THE TASK OF MEDICINE

THE TASK OF MEDICINE

DIALOGUE AT WICKENBURG

KERR L. WHITE, M.D.

THE HENRY J. KAISER FAMILY FOUNDATION
MENLO PARK, CALIFORNIA
1988

ISBN 0-944525-05-9

Library of Congress Catalogue Card Number: 87–82819

Design: Peter Rutledge Koch with the assistance of Eric Johnson. Printed in the United States of America

FOREWORD

THE PREVAILING PARADIGM that has shaped medical education, medical practices, and medical research for most of the twentieth century envisages disease as the end result of disordered molecular and biochemical processes. Such processes lead to cellular, tissue, organ, and system disturbance or destruction, resulting in disease, a characteristic constellation of specific biochemical, physiological and pathological anomalies. These anomalies are responsible for the specific loss of physical and other functions experienced by the patient and observed by the physician.

Dissatisfaction with the prevailing paradigm as a complete explanation of disease and illness has arisen in the past couple of decades. Coming largely from behaviorists, a broadened paradigm of medicine has emerged out of the certain knowledge that one disease may be manifest among a group of patients in widely divergent ways and that illness as experienced by patients may be as highly individualized as fingerprints. The modern paradigm, not by any means intended by its protagonists to replace but rather to broaden prevailing thought, interacts disease with personal, social and psychological factors to explain individual differences in illness. Despite face and experiential validity, the broadened paradigm has not achieved wide acceptance.

Nonetheless, patients often are not fully satisfied with the discourse in their physician's office and seem to say that their symptoms have not been satisfactorily explained. Some physicians, teachers and medical students also express concern with the prevailing paradigm. While probing opportunities for foundation attention we asked Charles Odegaard, Ph.D. to share his views, honed over nearly fifty years, on the current paradigm and its broadened modification. *Dear Doctor*, published by the Foundation in 1986, was one result.

Following *Dear Doctor* we asked Professor Odegaard to arrange a three-day conference of experts on these issues. The conference was held at the Wickenburg Inn, Wickenburg, Arizona on May 12–15, 1987. Kerr White, M.D., also having worked nearly a half century examining knowledge on the work of medicine, was asked to interpret the discussions at Wickenburg and to provide his personal thoughts on the underlying intellectual basis for medical practice. *The Task of Medicine, Dialogue at Wickenburg*, is one result.

Taking license from Dr. White's example I wish to add a personal thought to this volume. Although the broadened paradigm is an important and highly useful advance in medical thought, I believe it remains insufficiently broad for more effective medical practices given the current state of knowledge. A broad range of social, cultural and economic factors, nearly everything around us, importantly influence the state of health of individuals and nations. These influences include education, income level, racial and class status in society, customs and habits, advertising and other commercial practices, and the laws and regulations by which we are governed. These external factors, we now know, can have influences at any one point or on many points along the chain of events in the prevailing paradigm: biochemical, cellular and system function; disease onset and course; individual illness response; level of functioning in everyday activities; psychological state; and response to therapy. Knowledge of these external factors and their effects on individual health should be incorporated into a revised intellectual foundation for medicine.

It might be useful, therefore, to consider the paradigm of medicine to be in a never-finished state, in need of continued revision, and forever holding new promise for improving health and for enhancing physician effectiveness. The Dialogue at Wickenburg is *en route* to something better.

Alvin R. Tarlov, M.D.
President
Henry J. Kaiser Family Foundation

INTRODUCTION

SOCIETY'S STRUGGLES with the ills besetting heart and flesh did not start when the current medical establishment took office. To place American medicine's contemporary turmoil in perspective, however, it has required a professor of medieval history who, as a university president, once had a medical school in his bailiwick. And it has required a foundation officer, who as a professor of internal medicine acquired the "right" credentials, to initiate a national dialogue about the topics raised. Between them they have legitimized a critical review and discussion of the facts about the so-called "facts" as they bear on the problems and issues that define the profession's task and determine its priorities. These priorities should transcend the ephemeral quick fixes of the times and their focus on such epiphenomena as fiddling with payment schemes, hospital mergers, computer diagnosis and specialists' turf battles.

How can we agree on the qualitative and quantitative boundaries of the task of medicine as we respond to the needs of both individuals and society? What data and evidence do we need to establish the boundaries? What information and knowledge do we need to understand our task? How do we set about obtaining that information? If the heart of science and scholarship in any field is characterized by the nature and quality of the evidence, how do we establish the types, reliability and validity of evidence that medicine needs? Whose responsibility is it to take the lead? Who decides? Never forgetting that although information may be the starting point, it is, as T. S. Eliot reminds us, wisdom we seek. "Where is the wisdom we have lost in knowledge? Where is the knowledge we have lost in information?" (Eliot 1963).

At the invitation of Alvin R. Tarlov, President of the Henry J.

I

Kaiser Family Foundation, Charles Odegaard, forty physicians and four of their colleagues (Appendix VII) gathered at The Wickenburg Inn, Wickenburg, Arizona, May 12–15, 1987 for a *Conference on the Biopsychosocial Concept of Illness and Disease.* The point of departure was *Dear Doctor: A Personal Letter to a Physician,* Charles Odegaard's widely acclaimed volume on the historical origins of American medicine's unhappy bondage within its own constricted views of science and the human condition (Odegaard 1986). His monograph was augmented by a series of commissioned papers and published reprints circulated before the Conference, which were elaborated in oral presentations by the authors and discussed extensively, both formally and informally, during the Conference. Five of the commissioned papers and Dr. Odegaard's remarks initiating the dialogue are included in the present volume (Appendices I–VI).

The Conference was both an opportunity to reflect on the far-reaching insights provided by *Dear Doctor* and a challenge by the Kaiser Family Foundation for physicians themselves to initiate this national dialogue. As a basis for more clearly defining the task of medicine, the Conference focused primarily on the central role of the patient-physician relationship in both eliciting and communicating information—information essential for the medical profession to cope effectively with individual and collective needs and for medical schools to fulfill their missions.

My response to the invitation to write this essay combines two perspectives. The first attempts to capture the flavor as well as the substance of both the formal and, perhaps more importantly, the informal discussions at the Conference. The second attempts to follow Dr. Tarlov's injunction to "read between the lines," to "go beyond the explicit" and to express my "own views on a future agenda for medical education." In neither case have I followed the precise organization or sequence of presentations at the Conference. Rather, I have tried to summarize and expand on what seemed to me to be the central problems and issues raised in *Dear Doctor,* the circulated documents and the discussions at Wickenburg within a framework that could be readily understood by both physicians and non-physicians.

At the outset, however, it does seem important to be clear

that, apart from the central historical and cultural issues raised by Dr. Odegaard, virtually all of the problems and issues discussed at the Conference and much of the evidence have been voiced in medical circles for a long time—at least a generation. Therefore, to expand our historical base for understanding the profession's present confused state, I have tried to cite references and add evidence not used in the original Conference documents. In some instances when reflecting on the deliberations at Wickenburg, I have foreshortened arguments and omitted evidence that is well covered either in *Dear Doctor*, in the other papers and the Appendices of this volume, or in their excellent bibliographies.

In the final sections, the many different courses of action and potential change mentioned either formally or informally in the course of our deliberations have been combined with some thoughts of my own and consolidated into several generic initiatives. For all these liberties of interpretation and presentation I am responsible; I can only urge those who have not done so to read *Dear Doctor*, its appendices and the remaining papers in this volume. For those who wish to explore the issues further I have marked with an asterisk references for this essay that I have found stimulating.

PHYSICIAN AND PROFESSIONAL
PERSPECTIVES

As MIGHT BE ANTICIPATED, virtually all the Conference participants agreed that medicine needs to broaden its theoretical and
conceptual frameworks for considering the genesis and management of health and medical problems beyond the biological.
What is currently referred to as the biomedical model was seen
as extraordinarily useful but, at the same time, unduly restrictive. The narrow application of this model, clearly articulated by
Donald Seldin (Seldin 1981), and widely applauded by many academic leaders, can be taken as an honest description of the dominant intellectual perspective in the majority of contemporary
American medical schools:

> Medicine is a very narrow discipline. Its goals may be defined as the relief
> of pain, the prevention of disability, and the postponement of death by the
> application of the theoretical knowledge incorporated in medical science to
> individual patients. (Seldin 1981)

Similarly, Marcia Angell's editorial in the *New England Journal
of Medicine*, concluding that "it is time to acknowledge that our
belief in disease as a direct reflection of mental state is largely
folklore" (Angell 1985), may be an equally straightforward
comment stemming from the prevailing biomedical model
based on Cartesian dualism and the monoetiological or seventeenth century approach to understanding the origins of disease.

Most participants at the Wickenburg Conference would probably have agreed that both Seldin's and Angell's interpretations
of medicine's task are unduly narrow. They distort many of the
clinical realities of medical practice as perceived by a growing
number of physicians, large numbers of their patients and numerous scholars and scientists outside the medical establishment. The view that there are direct, one-to-one, linear etiolog-

4

ical links between reified "mental" and "disease" states has had few adherents over the years. Nevertheless, that has not prevented the biomedical model from being invoked frequently to dismiss what associative or interactive evidence does exist for the influence of psychological and social, or behavioral, to use a generic term now in widespread use, factors on health and disease.

The leading contender as a successor to the biomedical concept is often referred to by the awkward term, the biopsychosocial model (Engel Appendix II). Although the model's original formulation is appropriately associated with George Engel's work, the unfortunate label has been erroneously attributed to him. Over the years, this off-putting piece of jargon does not seem to have increased understanding or broadened acceptance. When the model itself is reified, contrasted with the biomedical model, and taught as a separate subject, seventeenth century dualism seems to be perpetuated rather than dissipated. To emphasize the substance of the arguments and the evidence advanced by the participants at Wickenburg and others it seems preferable to avoid, as much as possible, the term "biopsychosocial," and to speak of "expanded," "broader" or "more inclusive" theories or concepts of health and disease and even, as Dr. Engle suggested, of the "twentieth century" model in contrast to the "seventeenth century" model.

In Europe, Marco J. DeVries, Professor of Pathology at Erasmus University, Rotterdam, has advanced similar formulations in a remarkable little monograph, *The Redemption of the Intangible in Medicine* (1981). More recently, the World Health Organization Regional Office for Europe has published an excellent compendium of scholarly essays that bear on the models which guide the health care enterprise, *Scientific Approaches to Health and Health Care* (1986).

Whatever terminology we use in pursuing the national debate, there is every reason to take full cognizance of all the available evidence bearing on the desirability of broadening the search beyond the biological for information and knowledge related to the origins or our patients' illnesses. The case for this was well made in a substantial study conducted by the National

5

Academy of Science's Institute of Medicine, *Health and Behavior: Frontiers of Research in the Biobehavioral Sciences* (Hamburg, Elliott, and Parron 1982). Although not referred to at the Wickenburg Conference, many of the relationships, opportunities and problems addressed by the participants are discussed in the IOM study; in addition the report provides extensive bibliographies which should be helpful to those interested in fundamental and applied research that can contribute to this dialogue. In the face of this evidence, as well as that contained in the papers discussed at Wickenburg, we need to ask why medicine has been so slow in acting to implement and increase this knowledge. Why do we continue to behave as if it did not exist?

General system theory, of which the twentieth century model is a derivative, has been widely adopted by many scientific and technological disciplines and by many human organizations since von Bertalanffy first formulated it a generation ago (1951). And yet in the intervening decades, in spite of the acceptance of homeostasis as a biological concept, there has been little extension of cybernetic and systems thinking with their circular feedback loops to other hierarchies of understanding beyond the molecular, cellular and organ levels.

Nor has there been much change over the past half century in the central assumptions and concepts that guide the American medical enterprise. The need for a wider spectrum of premises, hypotheses and methods, and for greater specificity and clarity in defining them, in order to broaden medicine's horizons was enunciated clearly in the essay prepared for the Wickenburg Conference by Michael Schwartz and Osborne Wiggins (Appendix III). Their ideas were widely discussed but not universally accepted by the Conference participants. With helpful examples they urge that physicians strive to understand the everyday settings and circumstances in which their patients live and disease arises—their "lifeworlds." Apples are red and sweet as well as being composed of cells and molecules. A wave from a neighbor across the street is seen as "psychophysiologically neutral" because the observer does not distinguish between his friend's mental state and his motor functions.

Dr. Engle drew our attention to the recent publication of an important new work: *The Second Medical Revolution: From Biomedicine to Infomedicine* by Laurence Foss and Kenneth Rothenberg (1987). I would agree, it is a seminal work and a potentially major new contribution to the national dialogue initiated at Wickenburg. In this tightly argued and thoroughly documented volume the authors use principles derived from general system theory, information theory and artificial intelligence. They discuss the enormous potential for understanding health and disease that could stem from applying these ideas together with a wide spectrum of new extra-somatic information to develop an expanded model of health and disease—a model that does nothing to diminish the power or utility of biomedicine and much to enhance it. The following brief excerpt suggests the scope of the authors' thesis:

> The goal of the infomedical model can be generalized briefly as the accumulation of two levels of cybernetic understanding. The first level is to understand the 'programs' or 'grammar' that govern the interactions of the internal workings of the patient-as-cybernetic-system. Here, the rules governing the interactions of the parts are modeled. The second level is to understand which messages 'inform' the system and the nature of this impact. To inform, in this context, means to shape or reshape—literally to in-form or re-form. Messages from one level of organization can reshape and be reshaped by messages from another level of organization. As such, messages cannot be understood in isolation. Therefore, one must take into account both the environment in which the message circulates and the state of the system. Interpreting these messages turns them into information that the doctor or patient can then use to counter the disease/illness state. (Foss and Rothenberg 1987)

Although Foss and Rothenberg's term "infomedicine" may eventually replace "biomedicine," it seems fruitless to debate terminology at the expense of examining more fundamental issues. We should not confuse the "name" with the "thing" or reify ideas that are still in process of formation. What is needed is a dynamic and flexible approach that both accommodates currently available information and encourages the search for new evidence, new information and new theories. The processes themselves, as well as our knowledge about those processes, for describing, assessing and integrating objective and subjective experiences with a wide range of phenomena are forever expanding. Why, therefore, should any group try to constrain these efforts, let alone denigrate them, especially in universities? And yet the history of science and scholarship is replete with unhappy examples of just that (Stevenson 1958).

The formal organization and interpretation of human experience as a guide to action may have started with the Ionian Greeks. They probably originated the notion that qualitative differences in phenomena may be expressed mathematically—a development that grew apace with Galileo and later Newton. Although Aristotle contributed to this line of reasoning, he also emphasized the importance of observation and induction as a basis for generalization. Unfortunately his approach invoked too many "first principles" which were later found to be wrong. Francis Bacon challenged all this by calling for an end to prejudices and preconceptions about the nature of man and his surroundings. Bacon proposed combining induction with experimentation and deductive reasoning based on the rigorous testing of theories, especially those bearing on material matters. The negative ramifications stemming from this advance towards more critical and structured enquiry into man and his nature and man and his works are examined extensively in *Dear Doctor*.

What exactly, then, is science all about—especially as it bears on man's health and disease? Is the object of a scientific exercise restricted to collecting evidence to support or verify a theory? Is it to design an experiment to test the theory? Or is it to design an experiment to refute the theory as Karl Popper has advocated (Popper 1961)? The logic of the latter's position, which appears to include abandoning induction, has seemed inadequate to many. More acceptable has been Thomas Kuhn's notion of a paradigm shift (Kuhn 1970). This is said to occur when a body of accumulated evidence no longer fits the prevailing theory and a new theory must be invoked or induced, e.g., relativity and quantum physics as an extension of Newtonian physics and evolution as an extension of creationism. These shifts in the underlying concepts or theories usually take place at the periphery rather than centrally and are more apt to be acknowledged in retrospect than concurrently. When observations are inconsistent with the received formulations about the way things work, the theory or model tends to be misapplied to detract from or ignore the new facts. In turn, new concepts or theories are apt to be misrepresented as claiming to explain more than the evidence supports.

At least three factors seem to have contributed to much of contemporary academic medicine's allegedly restricted view of human health and disease. First, as Dr. Odegaard so eloquently sets forth, is the medical profession's widespread ignorance not only of its own history and the history of science but of the humanities generally. The collective contributions of those working in the humanistic tradition to appreciating and understanding expressions of the human condition in their infinite variety over time and place have been, too often, ignored. At Wickenburg there was a recognition, at least by some, of the extent of contemporary American medicine's intellectual poverty and of its unfortunate isolation from vast stores of wisdom and knowledge in other spheres of learning and experience beyond the biomedical.

Although C. P. Snow had drawn attention to the tragic separation of scientific and humanistic scholarship as a general academic problem in his Rede Lecture (Snow 1959), he emphasized its specific implications for medicine in his essay for the American Medical Association on "Human Care" (Snow 1973). Snow holds that physicians are unlikely to achieve their individual and collective potentials until there is full appreciation and understanding of both cultures. One of Snow's specific recommendations, and one with which Dr. Odegaard probably would have little quarrel, was that "there ought to be a literary component throughout the course of medical education." He went on to say, "this is a practical example of what I meant when I first spoke of the two cultures."

Those who would invoke Flexner to defend an exclusionary view are well-advised to consult a volume less frequently read by medical academicians than his "Report on Medical Education." Flexner wrote, as Dr. Odegaard reminds us, that:

. . . scientists—medical as well as other—owe something to themselves as human beings, something to the traditions and heirlooms of history, something to the unity and integrity of all science . . . [E]ven though a

issue. This is often psychologically impossible for experimental scientists. The more successful you get at manipulating (or apparently manipulating) theories, the harder it is not to believe in them.

Anti-realism flourishes in the counter-intuitive world of sub-atomic physics. (The Economist 1987)

To the last statement one can only ask, as Engel, DeVries, Schwartz and Wiggins, and Foss and Rothenberg might, "How can we encourage what some might regard as the twentieth century 'anti-realists' to flourish in medicine?" Granting the psychological impediments to modifying scientists' theories, and even the twentieth century theory itself, they are not insurmountable, as the revolutions in molecular biology, immunology, genetics and the neurosciences clearly demonstrate.

And a third factor contributing to academic medicine's restricted view is the notion that the development of technology based on scientific understanding and the deployment of that technology constitute science. To put it more bluntly, the emphasis in much narrowly defined biomedical research, particularly in clinical departments in recent decades, has been on "know how," rather than on "know why," "know whether" and "know what." Ever more elaborate descriptions of disease processes at the molecular, cellular, and organ levels and development of ever more complex interventions have been of unquestionable benefit. But explaining a process is not necessarily synonymous with understanding the origins of a phenomenon. In too many teaching environments, concern with improving skills in instrumentation appears to take precedence over efforts to expand the information base for clinical understanding and reasoning, and for patient counseling and management.

The proponents of the expanded model of health and disease argue for a much broader framework in which to understand the intricate and multifaceted web of causality that gives rise to our medical and related problems. Aristotle argued that the proper study of mankind was man; he did not argue that it was the compartmentalized study of molecular biology, immunology, psychiatry, anthropology, pharmacology, gastroenterology, or biochemistry. Somehow, it is argued, the primary focus of inquiry has to be redirected to individuals and their problems as they perceive them, with extensions down to the molecular and cellular levels and up to the interpersonal and societal levels, as the problems or questions require. People have problems; universities and governments seem to create ever more isolated departments!

But other than bemoaning the current turmoil in which the profession finds itself, there appear to be few among the American medical establishment who recognize the need for any major shift in priorities with respect to the content of medical education, as distinguished from changes in pedagogic ways and means. In the recent *Report of the Panel on the General Professional Education of the Physician and College Preparation for Medicine* (GPEP 1984) the preoccupations are with "how to teach" rather than with "what to learn." Proposals are scarce for new ways to select and change priorities in medical education and research and for new ways to organize the practice environment in which both take place.

Apart from the ill-fated war on cancer, nothing approaching such major interdisciplinary exercises as the Manhattan Project, NASA's space program or the short-lived boost in our educational efforts following Sputnik's launch, has even been contemplated as medicine's response to the intellectual, scientific and economic revolution engulfing our entry into the information age. There are those who argue that society's daunting contemporary health problems now merit at least as much innovative scientific and scholarly dedication as the earlier national initiatives. If not undertaken in the name of improving the human condition, they should then be discussed in the crass interests of long-term reductions in medical care expenditures, malpractice litigation and in government regulations—all reflections of massive societal discontent and discordance between medicine's and society's perceptions of the task.

Three distortions were identified by the Conference participants as contributing to sequestration of scientific and scholarly knowledge bearing on the expanded twentieth century model. The first has to do with the nature of evidence. In a court of law, at the human or personal level, reports of experiences, expressions of feelings and descriptions of events are accepted as evidence after cross examination, triangulation and confirmation; not so in medicine. Patients' views of their problems, complaints, and symptoms and their own theories about possible relationships to the life they lead are given short shrift. If the phenomenon can be measured or counted it is regarded as being more credible and useful than if it is observed, reported or even experienced, regardless of its intrinsic contribution to understanding or explaining the matter at hand (Ziman 1978).

Examples abound, but one mentioned at Wickenburg was the report of a new "disease": Liqueur lung (Conette et al. 1987). An otherwise healthy young man complained that he coughed up a cup of blood. He was subjected to several thousand dollars worth of tests including an uncomfortable examination of his lungs with a bronchoscope and biopsy of lung tissue. All findings were normal. These findings, the authors stated, "prompted additional questioning of the patient." Whereupon he told them that he had "been at a party and had guzzled from a bottle of Bucca." While drinking in this manner he began to choke and cough repeatedly and a few hours later he spat up blood. So far have we gone in denying the utility of information about the patient and his problems that is not derived from laboratory studies and instrumentation that, apparently, in at least some medical circles, an initial history of the presenting illness is no longer considered necessary.

Gayle Stephen's moving essay (Appendix IV) reminds us that first and foremost it is trust, communication, appreciation and understanding that are more often than not the necessary, if not always sufficient, requirements for obtaining the information essential to care for one another. Desirable as measuring and counting are, they are not substitutes for other standards of validity, reliability, accuracy and utility. Evidence to be used in scientific evaluations must surely be judged more on the basis of its credibility, reproducibility and generalizability than on the basis of any numbers that may be associated with it. As Michael Schwartz and Osborne Wiggins argue cogently, the latter are usually only proxies or codes to assist in comparing abstractions of the underlying phenomena (Appendix III).

The scientific method should be as much concerned with the

For Isabel – who understands so much.

CONTENTS

observer as it is with the subject observed. Hence in its application, high priority is given to identifying and accounting for biases, observer errors and variations of all types—and even values. To suggest that science, medicine or medical research is value-free is to ignore reality and experience; some questions or problems must be "valued" more than others by the investigator, the teacher or the physician, if not by the public.

Science is as much concerned with defining and classifying as it is with counting. Medical science is as much concerned with listening and observing as it is with measurement. Medicine deals not only with molecules, cells, and organs but also with people—individually and collectively. Even reified abstractions reflect some underlying phenomena. As Major Greenwood, the eminent British statistician, used to say, "health statistics represent people—people with the tears wiped off!"

The second distortion, related to the first, concerns the quaint notion in many medical circles that measurement, usually in some linear mode, is the be all and end all of the scientific enterprise. Interested as I have been over the years in improving clinicians' capacities for critical appraisal of evidence of all types through improved "numeracy," we should all be clear that measurement is simply one, but far from the only, way of dealing with bias and error of many types. It is a shorthand or proxy for describing the underlying phenomenon, as Alvan Feinstein, one of the prime movers in introducing clinicians to the concepts and methods of epidemiology, argues forcibly in a recent scholarly article. He writes:

> . . . clinicians have searched for 'hard' data, preferably expressed in the dimensional numbers of laboratory measurements. The consequence has been a deliberate reduction of the human information used in clinical science. The data obtained from personal observations and clinical judgment have often been rejected as too 'soft' to be worthy of scientific attention.
>
> Among the soft information excluded by this model are data about a patient's spectrum of symptoms, severity of illness, co-morbidity, disability, and all the distinctly human reactions—love, hate, joy, sorrow, distress, gratification—that differentiate people from animals or molecules. The exclusions have also diverted attention from the clinician's traditional obligation to offer relief and comfort, not just cure. Consequently, the results of treatment today are often reported with hard data about death,

15

survival, disease, and adverse reactions, but suitable information is not assembled to show many important human benefits of modern therapy.

> For the challenges of a new humanistic clinical science, the soft data that describe distinctive clinical and human phenomena must be hardened and made intellectually respectable. (Feinstein 1987)

Although measurement is highly desirable for manipulating many kinds of evidence, not everything that is measured is important and not everything that is important can be measured, at least with the concepts and methods currently available. Measurement is not the same as comparison, however. Much evidence, including that produced from biomedical investigations, is susceptible to measurement by interval scales. There are other phenomena, especially those derived from clinical experience, that are susceptible to other means of comparison widely used by social scientists and even by historians but which have not been fully exploited in medicine. Frederick Mosteller and his colleagues describe these in a volume that should be read by all physicians who aspire to be scientists, *Data for Decisions*; the entire volume has five simple tables and five equations but admirably covers the diverse ways of eliciting, arraying and assessing evidence of many types (Hoaghlin et al. 1982). In matters of clinical judgment as well as public policy it is usually better to be roughly right than precisely wrong!

Some phenomena are best named or labeled first, then classified and compared using nominal scales. Others are more susceptible to comparison by ranking in an ordinal scale and still others are best expressed in relationships using ratio and other scales, pattern recognition and a wide variety of indexes. Beyond these are other observations and experiences that can only be described and not a few of the latter that were only "felt." Measurement, desirable though it may be as an adjunct to many applications of the scientific method, is not nearly as important as clear and logical thinking (Ziman 1978). At Wickenburg, Drs. Schwartz and Wiggins put the issue succinctly:

> . . . [P]recision and exactitude are not essential requirements of science. Faithfulness to the evidence within the critical attitude is the essential requirement of scientific activity. (Appendix III)

In the final analysis, however, comparison is usually the critical maneuver as demonstrated daily by wine tasters and livestock judges.

The third distortion results from medicine, often regarded as the mother of science and the base from which man and his ills are best studied, having lost many of its central features during the nineteenth century. Previously clinical medicine usually had been synonymous with all of "medicine" as scholars and scientists sought better explanation and understanding of disease first through the study of morbid anatomy and later of physiology, microbiology and their derivative disciplines. As a result of the unquestioned productivity stemming from the pursuit of these branches of science they acquired the collective appellation "basic." In turn, supported by the prevailing notions, extensions of the seventeenth century model, that man and his nature are best explained in terms of the even more fundamental sciences of physics, chemistry and biology, they grew in stature and influence.

Bolstered by selective reading and repetition to each other of some of Flexner's views, these major preclinical, natural science disciplines have, especially since World War II, expanded and flourished in the United States and to a large extent in other Western industrialized countries. Indeed the derivative basic disciplines seem to have taken on a life of their own in medical schools. Some would say that, however remarkably they may have contributed to our explanation of fundamental processes, their knowledge base is often only indirectly related to many of the individual and collective tasks of medicine as a practicing profession. At the same time, other scientific investigators and scholars have languished, though perhaps with an equal or even better claim on the term "basic," but using other types of evidence and other sites and populations for their inquiries. Again, as Dr. Odegaard has urged, let us listen to Flexner:

> In what sense, then, can modern medicine today be called a science? If the term "science" is to be strictly confined to knowledge capable of quantitative expression and utilization, science would begin and end with mathematical physics—itself perhaps not of the final character supposed in the days before the coming of Einstein; chemistry and physiology would be

sciences, insofar as they are reducible to physics and no further. Other disciplines, to which we now attach the name—the social sciences, for example, or agriculture, in which an increasing volume of systematized knowledge and practical art is, as in medicine, indistinguishably blended—would cease to be so called.

Neither on theoretical nor on practical grounds can so narrow a use of the term be successfully defended. We do better, taking an historical view, to consider science as the persistent effort of men to purify, extend, and organize their knowledge of the world in which they live. Undoubtedly the more accurately—or mathematically—the organization of knowledge can proceed, the better; and mathematical form may well be recognized as the goal towards which scientific effort strives. *But it is absurd* (emphasis added) to set up the single mathematical category, which ignores complications of material that may prove forever refractory, or innate limitations of capacity beyond which men cannot go. For practical purposes, at any rate, science must be considered as simply the severest effort capable of being made in the direction of purifying, extending, and organizing knowledge. So long as men strive to transcend their native powers, to rid themselves of prejudice and preconception, to observe phenomena in a dry light, the effort is scientific. How much success the effort must achieve, how large a volume of fact must have been accumulated and set in order, how far laws must be deduced, before one is entitled to speak of a science rather than of scientific effort—these are questions that permit of no invariable answer. (Flexner 1925)

By clinging to a seventeenth century model of health and disease American academic medicine has been able to apply with enormous success some features of the scientific method to a limited set of phenomena bearing on selected aspects of health and disease. At the same time we seem to have learned little or nothing about many other manifestations of health and disease. We have yet to apply the full range of scientific and humanistic thought and methods to understand more fully medicine's role in the larger scheme of human affairs or even to help us in defining our collective task. We do not seem to understand that not only other physicians, but also many other scholars and scientists with diverse interests, have gone before and have considered the problems and issues we still ponder and have advanced rather different formulations for understanding and appreciating them. For all of this, the contemporary version of the seventeenth century biomedical model is seen as inadequate, useful as it may be for explaining many of the molecular and cellular subsystems participating in the complex processes associated with health and disease.

Biomedicine bashing was not in evidence at the Conference. There was no suggestion from any source that developments ensuing from application of the biomedical model should not be encouraged in every way possible. Since World War II there have been unquestionable advances in our understanding of many of the processes and causal factors that influence health and disease. We have had a spate of efficacious interventions stemming directly from fundamental biomedical and population-based research; and there is much more to come. That is not really at issue. To suggest that the biomedical model may have limitations in no way diminishes the achievements of the past or the potential for the future. It is to suggest, however, that there may be broader and more inclusive ways of looking at individual and collective problems of health and disease that may also prove fruitful—and in the experience of many of the Conference participants, clinically helpful.

What is needed, first and foremost throughout academic medicine, as Eisenberg (Appendix V) and the Institute of Medicine study (Hamburg, Elliott, and Parron 1982) argue, is more, not less, and broader, not narrower, scientific thinking and scholarship. In addition, there is a need for more and different types of integration and interaction with those sciences that Flexner's disciples excluded from the medical arena. These include experimental psychology, anthropology, sociology, demography, economics, epidemiology, health statistics—the behavioral and population-based sciences. We need to encourage linkages among wet-laboratory scientists, clinical investigators studying individual patients, and those studying populations in communities.

Joseph Needham, the eminent biologist, wrote 50 years ago that this issue is:

> . . . by no means of purely philosophical interest, for if we take an organism belonging to one of the higher levels (such as a rabbit or an archbishop) we are only too aware that we make progress in our understanding of it, not by confining our studies to one level, such as psychological or chemi-

cal, but attacking its analysis at all levels, and then putting the results together at the level of imaginative synthesis. And here comes the root of the trouble, for the union of the sciences is much easier to talk about than to put into practice. (Needham 1936)

Although there are examples of such linkages here and there, they have been, as Needham implied, the exception rather than the rule. Certainly there has been no recent large-scale formal shift in the focus of medicine's task commensurate in direction or scale with that which followed the Flexner Report and the introduction of the natural sciences into medical schools. The GPEP Report does not seem to recognize, to say nothing of grapple with, many of these central problems.

Even among the participants at Wickenburg there also appeared to be scant familiarity with what had been done by earlier cohorts of medical academicians to address the problems discussed. Our contemporary medical establishment seems unaware that during the twentieth century, in addition to the revolution in molecular biology, a variety of different, expanded, and more inclusive models have emerged and that criticisms of the Flexnerian model are not of recent origin. Sir James Mackenzie is one of the great heroes of family physicians because of his research on the prognostic meaning of patients' signs and symptoms. On the basis of meticulous observations of his patients in their natural habitats he became the preeminent cardiologist of his day. The author of numerous textbooks and monographs that revolutionized cardiology, he also wrote several volumes on medical education and research that are almost timeless (Mackenzie 1919). In 1919 on an extended visit to the United States he questioned the truncated nature of the Flexnerian revolution. He appears to have had grave reservations about the emerging theoretical underpinnings for medical education, research and practice in America when, after visiting Baltimore, he wrote:

. . . the Johns Hopkins School was reckoned to be in the very forefront of medical schools, having enormous endowments, so that medicine is broken up into a great number of specialities, and the students have to learn an enormous number of different methods, but in conversation with the authorities, I never was more surprised to find such a stupid outlook as they possessed. I could say with confidence, that we were far better taught in Edinburgh in our days than the men [sic] are today in such places. But what struck me above all, was their absolute conceit and complacence, and when we discussed certain phases of medicine in which they pretended to being the most up-to-date, I found them extraordinarily superficial. So far as my own work is concerned, they had not even realized the elementary principles necessary to guide them in understanding the meaning of symptoms which their numerous methods revealed. (Mair 1973)

About the same time Jan Smuts wrote extensively about the philosophical and scientific concept of holism (Smuts 1926), a concept which many of those disenchanted with some aspects of contemporary orthodox medicine find attractive today. A decade later the highly imaginative Peckham Experiment in London initiated a long-term research strategy to test some of the hypotheses derived from observing the manifestations of health and disease in families living in their natural habitats (Pearse and Crocker 1943 and Pearse 1979). Many other examples could be cited, such as the longitudinal studies using expanded biological, psychological and social models initiated in the forties and fifties in Aberdeen (Scotland), Alameda County (California), Baltimore, Boston, Claxton County (Georgia), Denver, Framingham, Newcastle (England), London and Tecumseh (Michigan), to mention only some of the better known sites.

And then there were the intensive but short-lived educational forays into "comprehensive medicine" sponsored by the Commonwealth Fund in the 1950s (Lee 1962). Indeed, as described, demonstrated and advocated at Wickenburg, many of the attitudes towards patients, skills in interviewing, integrated, general or "comprehensive" clinics and longitudinal care and follow-up of patients and their families, were all well-developed during that period in at least nine major medical schools. That a number of the younger Conference participants spent time at one or more of those schools suggests that the flames may not have been entirely extinguished by the extraordinary achievements of biomedicine. During much of this era Dr. Engle's influence was emerging as he formulated and refined his model and trained all too few to follow in his footsteps (Appendix II).

Alas, the impact has been modest compared to the wonders wrought by the molecular revolution. But a revolution in one system does not an entire systems revolution make!

Awareness of contemporary activities in various academic camps also was lacking among many participants at Wickenburg. Specifically, the general internists and the family physicians seemed to know little about each other's interests or agendas. For example: there is the Society of Teachers of Family Medicine's Family Practice Faculty Development Institutes conducted for many years by the Baylor University College of Medicine's Center for Medical Education at Waco, Texas; the fifteen-year-old North American Primary Care Research Group (Wood 1981); the six-year-old Ambulatory Sentinel Practice Network (Green, Wood, Becker et al. 1984); and the work underway in Divisions of General Internal Medicine on interviewing (Lipkin, Quill, and Napodano 1984), clinical decision-making, critical appraisal, and design, measurement and evaluation (Fletcher, Fletcher, and Wagner 1982 and Sackett, Haynes, and Tugwell 1985).

There is, indeed, a wealth of knowledge and experience that could be shared among medical academicians of all persuasions. Sharing is also essential among physicians and their fellow scholars and scientists in other sectors of the wider university community to understand better those dimensions of the human condition that find expression as pain, suffering and disability. One purpose of the Conference was to lower these barriers, place our collective efforts in historical perspective and initiate a national dialogue; in this the Conference seemed remarkably successful.

Since World War II both the academic and administrative medical establishments in the United States have ignored implicitly, if not explicitly, the need for elaborating a more inclusive theory of health and disease. Substantial amounts of scientific, clinical, anecdotal and popular evidence in support of the need for an expanded model have been accumulating. Compared to the magnificent research accomplishments stemming from application of the biomedical model, pursuit of a more inclusive twentieth century model seemed to have precious little to offer.

Even in the halcyon days of unfettered medical research budgets there were relatively few systematically designed analyses and experiments at either the macro, i.e., the population level, or at the micro, i.e., the individual and cellular levels, to examine the validity and, as necessary, to suggest revisions of the underlying theory. Indeed, it is not unfair to say, as Kuhn predicted, that most of the leaders of the contemporary medical establishment, especially its academic component, have rejected not only the theory but also the available evidence.

There was broad consensus at the Conference that fundamental changes were in store for American academic medicine, but it was also argued that the first step was to increase awareness and understanding of the central problems medicine faces, the issues surrounding them, and their implications for medical education, practice, research and organization. Important as adoption of an expanded theory of health and disease may be, there was virtual unanimity among the participants that any acceptable theory bearing on the task of medicine should encompass the extraordinary insights stemming from the revolution wrought by advances in molecular biology, especially in genetics and immunology. Nor was there the slightest disposition to minimize those remarkable technological interventions developed in the last half century that are truly both efficacious and effective.

The central issue is whether, in addition to the phenomenal advances in biological aspects of medicine, there are other experiences, other kinds of evidence and information, other perspectives, other ways of thinking about the problems, and other interventions and maneuvers that could further enhance healing and the maintenance of health. More specifically, are there behavioral (i.e., psychological, attitudinal and social) factors that materially influence health and disease which deserve similar emphasis and attention?

Are there group, community and population factors, such as social and economic circumstances, in addition to individual, cellular and molecular influences that, if they do not harbor the seeds of another scientific revolution, might, if better understood and applied, materially enhance the progress made by biomedicine? The answer is "yes." For over thirty years, anthropologists, sociologists and epidemiologists have been documenting the impact of social, cultural and economic factors on the origins of disease and the outcomes of measures to ameliorate them (Jaco 1958).

To what extent should the behavioral and population perspectives, in addition to the biological, be embraced in education, research and teaching to achieve a balanced understanding of health and disease? To what extent do observations and insights about emotional, cultural and social factors experienced in familial, domestic, neighborhood and occupational settings, for example, interacting among themselves while also interacting with genetic, nutritional, environmental factors help us to understand and cope with disease and illness? How do these relationships, long acknowledged by many physicians and large numbers of their patients, as well as by humanists and behavioral scientists, affect people's health? How can other kinds or new (i.e., new to the contemporary medical establishment) kinds of information and evidence best be garnered and applied in the course of individual physician-patient interactions and communications? And how can this new information best be used in the course of negotiating the social contract between the medical establishment and society so that it plays a central role in defining the task of medicine?

At the outset of our national dialogue we should be crystal clear that of all the things doctors, nurses and other health personnel currently do for patients, probably no more than 20 percent of their therapeutic interventions are supported by objective evidence that they do more good than harm (Eisenberg Appendix V). That, however, is an extraordinary achievement given the state of affairs a generation ago. Of equal importance is the observation that, on average, the ubiquitous placebo effect accounts for some 35 to 40 percent of clinical benefits (Brody 1980). The related, but probably discrete, Hawthorne effect accounts, on average, for about another 15 to 20 percent (Mayo 1933). Apparently about a quarter of all benefits are still a mystery! Too often physicians take the view that improvements in their patients' well-being, unassociated with a demonstrably efficacious intervention, are the result of "just the placebo or Hawthorne effects." Perhaps we should look at these combined phenomena, and the related ones of meditation and relaxation in another way and, as they did at a National Workshop in India, call them "Factor X", propose that they be investigated extensively, and look on them as the most powerful therapeutic agents in existence (Bisht 1985).

The doctor herself or himself may indeed be a prime mediator of that agent as Michael Balint argued (1955) and as Ian Mc-Whinney and his colleagues have demonstrated (Appendix VI). In a carefully designed study they have shown that the strongest predictors of the outcomes of patient care were the patient's report that he or she had been able to discuss the problem fully with the physician and the patient's complete agreement with the physician's opinion of the problem. Or as Adolf Meyer, the first professor of psychiatry at the Johns Hopkins Hospital, used to say, "When patient and doctor agree on the nature of the problem, the patient generally gets better!"

The nature of the evidence bearing on potentially sensitive psychological and social factors may constitute the barrier. Lack of familiarity with the methods for establishing the reliability and validity of new forms of evidence may be an obstacle. Is it possible that ignorance of the methods for reducing, manipulating and analyzing the data is a hindrance? Or is the problem poverty of experience and exposure? Has the contemporary biomedical scientist never been exposed to the vast sweep of human history? Is he or she unaware of our efforts to understand ourselves and our works in some broader context than abstractions viewed solely from the molecular and cellular perspectives—remarkably useful as they are for their specific purposes? If political and geographic history, biography, philosophy, the "novel as life," poetry, art and music have eluded many members of the contemporary medical establishment, then whatever happened to the philosophy and history of science, and the history of medicine itself? If these deficiencies could be overcome would it not be reasonable to expect that the testing of expanded theories of health and disease, commensurate with other achievements in twentieth century medical science, might ensue?

Some or all of these factors, in addition to the broader historical trends so fully described by Dr. Odegaard, must help to account for our present truncated perspective. How else does one explain the present medical establishment's rejection of evidence accumulated over 50 years that is incompatible with the seventeenth century biomedical model? Apparently there are those among us who missed, for example, Walter B. Cannon's work half a century ago on the influence of emotional factors on bodily function (Cannon 1932), who have forgotten Curt Richter's studies of the influence of "hope" on the survival time of rats and the implications of his findings for humans (1957), or who have chosen to ignore George Engel's own series of 170 deaths accompanying severe emotional trauma (1971). In spite of a rich descriptive and analytical literature, augmented by more limited experimental evidence, many in the current medical establishment appear unconvinced, scattered protestations to the contrary, that psychological, social and environmental factors have much to do with health and disease, merit vigorous investigation and should be discussed fully with patients and students.

In a poignant volume by David Hilfiker, *Healing the Wounds*, a Harvard medical student is quoted:

> I have already been horrified by the glaring lack of emphasis in the curriculum on the social and psychological aspects of medicine or the emotional stresses of being a physician. None of our professors is willing to discuss the feelings which the phenomenon of disease elicits in both patient and doctor. Only doctors who can provide 'miraculous' cures and patients who are cooperative and articulate are presented. There is no time to express our feelings of sadness for the patient, to articulate our fear that he or she or relatives or ourselves will die, to discuss the impact of our decision to enter a profession where suffering is a constant companion. Instead, we flounder, striving to ask insightful questions both to impress our instructors and to combat our sense of sadness and inadequacy. We are taught from the beginning not to express our emotions, as if they might in some way interfere with our ability to be competent doctors. Conflict is rarely presented; mistakes never mentioned. I often question whether I will be able to keep up with recent advances, or to stay alert during the long hours of residency and medical practice, or to understand and empathize with my patients, all of which are necessary to provide quality care. My medical training, by ignoring these questions, is not making me more confident about these issues, rather it is teaching me not to consider them, denying me the chance to recognize my fears. (Hilfiker 1985)

If discussion of individual patient's and individual student's emotional reactions to illness is too threatening, surely examination of these phenomena in the aggregate should be less distressing.

What, then, have the population-based sciences been telling us? For almost fifty years sociologists, anthropologists, demographers, epidemiologists and health statisticians have provided abundant evidence that unemployment, plant closings, recessions, deprivation, separations, widowhood, love and support, promotions, job changes, occupational mobility, divorces and other manifestations of the joys and sorrows that mark the struggle for survival take their tolls in human illness and impairments (Broadhead et al. 1983; Cassel, Patrick, and Jenkins 1960; Ciocco 1941; Hamburg, Elliott, and Parron 1982; Helsing, Comstock, and Szklo 1982; Moser, Fox, and Jones 1984).

Several examples will illustrate the potential contributions to be made by employing population-based methods to study the impact of these factors; two of them were discussed by their authors at Wickenburg. Jack Medalie's ground-breaking study of angina pectoris established the therapeutic power of love and support, especially when provided by the spouse, on survival (Medalie and Goldbourt 1976), findings which were supported in the related population-based study by Chandra et al. (1983). Next was Robert Haggerty's study done 25 years ago of the positive association between domestic strife and susceptibility to streptococcal infections (Haggerty 1987). Then there was the threefold increase in mortality associated with unannounced relocation of aged and disabled patients in nursing homes (Aldrich and Mendkoff 1963). Neale and Nethercott (1985) reported that in response to both the insecurity of an anticipated plant closing and the plant closing itself there was a substantial increase in visits to doctors and to hospital outpatient departments by those affected and by their families, compared to control populations. And more recently the latest of many other studies of the negative impact of unemployment on mortality demonstrates both the time lags and the selective effects involved (Forbes and McGregor 1987).

But these data are generated by the so-called "soft sciences"—

as if that were the issue. Those who work in wet laboratories of medical schools have tended to use the term "hard" science to characterize their own contributions and to assign the term "soft" science to those who work in the social and behavioral sciences. Surely the issue is not whether the data are obtained from a wet laboratory, a clinic or hospital or from a population. Surely it is not whether the evidence is derived from instrumental measurements of body fluids, from carefully triangulated, nondirective interviews with a patient and the family, or from household surveys, or the assessment of housing conditions. The issue is whether the information generated is credible, replicable and useful and whether the question or problem is approached with an inquiring, skeptical curiosity characterized by awe, wonder and humility. These are the qualities that make the effort scientific and scholarly. No one branch of science, and no one type of evidence has a monopoly on defining credibility. Even basic, and especially many clinical, scientific papers are flawed in their designs, methods, analyses or interpretations; there is much room for improvement in all branches of science (Bailar and Mosteller 1986).

The term "basic" when arrogated by one group of scientists seems to imply a measure of hubris in the face of the evidence. Who is to say which aspects of science and scholarship will, in both the short-term and the long-term, contribute most to improving the human condition? Which aspects of science will be regarded as fundamental to our understanding of health and disease when both the ever-expanding body of extra-somatic information is assimilated and the twentieth century model of health and disease is tested more aggressively and critically? Surely, as Arnold Toynbee is alleged to have said when asked for his views on the outcome of the French Revolution, "it's too soon to tell!"

Apart from *Dear Doctor* and the papers in the Appendices of this volume with their extensive bibliographies, at least two integrative works have assembled substantial amounts of the available descriptive, analytical and experimental evidence that really require for their understanding and explanation an expanded and more inclusive paradigm than the biomedical model. Robert Ader and his colleagues have set forth evidence that builds on the work of Cannon, Richter and even Hans Selye, of whom it was once alleged, "his facts may be wrong but his theories may be right!" This newly emerging interdisciplinary field of psycho-neuroimmunology bears yet another unfortunate label—like biopsychosocial, forced on us by the fragmentation of scientific disciplines—to designate a problem-oriented, integrated field of study (Ader and Cohen 1981). Although based on animal studies their work cannot be summarily disregarded, any more than evidence from more restricted biomedical animal studies can be dismissed or ignored by any even-handed scientific commentator. Similarly, Christian Ramsey and his colleagues have prepared a volume of what must be one of the most extensive reviews and syntheses of laboratory, clinical and population-based research extant that bear on the scientific underpinnings of the inclusive theory of health and disease considered at the Wickenburg Conference. Again, for want of more apt terminology, this intriguing volume is called *Family Systems in Medicine* (Ramsey 1988).

Although concern about theoretical concepts, terms and assumptions underlay all the discussions, they were not really what the Conference was all about. Rather, the operational focus was on the practical relationships of individual physicians with their patients and on the medical profession's collective relationships with society. By extension the Conference was concerned with the means by which medical students, residents, and even faculty might learn more about the complex transactions that govern those relationships. Within that context, most attention was paid to the kinds and credibility of the data, evidence, information and knowledge that could be garnered to further enlighten and guide the task of medicine. To gain some flavor of these concerns I turn now to a consideration of this task as it appears from the viewpoints of the individual and the population, i.e., society.

PATIENT AND POPULATION
PERSPECTIVES

THE CONFERENCE PARTICIPANTS brought diverse experiences and approaches to both the problems addressed and the solutions proposed. Nevertheless, a consensus seemed to emerge that change was needed and that now is the time to start. A sea change in society's and patients' attitudes and expectations of doctors, nurses, their colleagues, and their institutions is under way. Manifestations of that change include: the ending of medicine's conspiracy of silence and the outmoded illusion that "doctors know best" (Katz 1984); unwillingness on the part of patients and their families to tolerate further patient abuse (Stevenson 1985); the unseemly avalanche of medical malpractice litigation and the spate of wellness clinics and health spas—all with their associated gatherings, literature and acolytes.

To swell the waves of change there is the vulgar preoccupation on the part of both the public and their politicians with the ever increasing costs of the whole enterprise—and not just in money. The "be kind to patients" movement has its devotees and hospitals are enjoining all hands to smile at the customers in order to increase "market share." These may be all to the good and some may well constitute substantial improvements. Many, however, are epiphenomena churned up by the underlying currents and they too will pass!

This change in attitudes and expectations is at the root of the revolution in which medicine now finds itself—a revolution precipitated in part by the molecular and technological revolutions wrought by biomedicine and in part by our widespread failure to assimilate large amounts of extra-somatic or nonbiological experience and information.

One of the clearest manifestations of this revolution is the massive shift from a "supply" dominated model of medicine's task, controlled by the country's medical schools, to a "demand" dominated model based on the perceived needs and attributes of the individuals and populations served. Examples include the "Health for All by the Year 2000" movement initiated by UNICEF and the World Health Organization, the vertical integration of American health care arrangements by investor-owned corporations, and the hierarchical approaches to resource allocation and priorities in Sweden (Engel 1968) and Finland (Finnish Ministry of Social Affairs and Health 1985).

In the course of this shift the prevailing biomedical model, as well as the manpower, institutional and organizational arrangements it supports, is found wanting. A much broader view of both physician–patient and professional–societal relations is required if we are to fulfill medicine's task. As Dr. Odegaard emphasizes once again in his essay "Towards an Improved Dialogue" (Appendix I), this broader view requires that we appreciate fully our historical origins as both a learned profession and a scholarly endeavor directed at helping people.

Most participants at Wickenburg seemed to agree that there are fundamental problems with the conceptual and organizational underpinnings of contemporary American academic medicine that severely restrict it from reaching its full potential. Moreover, the seventeenth century model is seen as inhibiting many aspects of legitimate inquiry into each individual patient's problems and, as a consequence, into the population's priorities. These inquiries have the potential for expanding and enhancing contributions from the more limited biological perspective. The impact of the prevailing biotechnical view of health and disease on both the education of medical students and on the care of patients and populations in the view of at least some of the Conference participants is often counterproductive and may, at times, be destructive.

Examples abound. Tape and video recordings of patients in their first encounters with medical students and house staff and, one suspects, with many practicing physicians, still reflect the power struggle between the former trying to describe his or her problems and the latter trying to take a history. "Stop telling me about your problems and just answer the questions!" the physician, driven by a *furor therapeuticus*, is apt to say, while interrupting the patient a few seconds (18 by actual count, in a large series, according to one participant) after the interview starts. "If you ask questions, you get answers," Michael Balint wrote (1957). Why shouldn't the patient be allowed to set the agenda for the encounter, particularly when he or she is ambulatory, conscious, competent and footing the bill? Why shouldn't the capable patient establish the rules for the encounter, as Szasz and Hollender outlined in their classic article published the same year (1957)? Why shouldn't the dialogue be conducted in the patient's language rather than the medical profession's jargon? Why shouldn't all transactions be referred to what Schwartz and Wiggins call the patient's "lifeworld" or "lived body," rather than to the medical profession's abstractions (Appendix III)? It was reported at the Conference that a large-scale analysis of clinical records turned up less than one word per chart that reflected any concern for social and psychological factors bearing on the patient's illness. What type of doctor-patient relationship does this reflect? What kind of communications skill on the part of the physician does it suggest?

Over sixty years ago the first systematic treatise on the interview described it as "a conversation with a purpose" (Bingham and Moore 1924). Surely the central purposes for the physician when first interviewing a patient are to determine: (1) the nature and origins of the patient's problem as he or she defines it; (2) why the patient seeks care at this particular juncture; (3) why care is sought from this particular source; and (4) what the patient's theory is about the genesis of the problem. Forty-five years have passed since Carl Rogers introduced the "Uh-huh" or "What-else?" techniques of nondirective interviewing, perhaps the simplest and most effective means of conducting a "conversation with a purpose," in contrast to obtaining "answers" to "questions" (Rogers 1942). Thirty-five years have passed since Stewart Wolf published his volume on interviewing entitled *Talking with the Patient* (1952), thirty-two years since Brian Bird first published his volume *Talking with Patients* (Bird 1955) and Michael Balint first published his observations on "The Doctor, His Patient, and the Illness" (Balint 1955), and thirty years since Robert Kahn and Charles Cannell published their definitive work on the theory and practice of interviewing, including a section on medical interviewing (Kahn and Cannell 1957).

Twenty-seven years ago M. L. Johnson Abercrombie of the Department of Anatomy, University College, London, published her pioneering work on perception, information and reasoning in medicine. Her remarkable little volume is full of excellent exercises which still can be studied with profit by medical teachers. She discusses in considerable detail:

> . . . aspects of the relation between the inner and outer worlds, . . . emphasizes the selective and interpretative nature of perception, and shows how the information that a person gets from the outer world depends on the context, or total situation, and on his past experience, which is usefully thought of as being organized into schemata. Human relationships play an important role in perception both in that they are often a significant part of the context, and in that they have contributed to the formation, testing and modifying of schemata. (Abercrombie 1960)

In many respects Abercrombie made the logical case, as distinguished from the historical and humanitarian cases, for adopting the expanded, twentieth century, model. She would have been a valuable participant at Wickenburg.

The intervening decades have seen countless articles, manuals and books published on interviewing and on broadening the information base for medical decisions. Yet there is a persistent inability or unwillingness on the part of what is alleged to be a majority of physicians to converse, to listen, to try to understand, to learn about the patient's "lifeworld," the natural history of the illness and the search for help, and about the circumstances under which the illness arose and the meaning to the individual of his or her symptoms and illness. If this is not a medical disgrace it must be close to it. Indeed lack of interviewing and communication skills is probably the root cause of our malaise vis-à-vis the public and our patients.

Other helping professions such as lawyers, the clergy, social workers and nurses, for example, and those who work in service industries such as innkeeping, air transport, banking and retail selling, for example, seem to expend considerable effort on learning, honing and monitoring their communications and interviewing skills; but not physicians. Their communication skills must be at an all-time low; in the public's view, however, it would appear to be the physicians who need these skills most.

A new manual and a series of nationwide faculty workshops and associated courses on interviewing have been developed by a Task Force of the Society for General Internal Medicine (SGIM), formerly the Society for Research and Education in Primary Care Internal Medicine (SREPCIM) of the American College of Physicians, (Lipkin, Quill, and Napodana 1984). This is a highly laudable, timely, and even urgently needed undertaking given the present deplorable state of affairs. To those who have labored in the vineyard of patient-physician relationships and communication over the years, this effort has to be regarded in much the same way as remedial reading courses are for many contemporary high school and even college students. Although a necessary step in addressing our enormous problems, it is scarcely sufficient. Much more is needed.

Why do medical schools stifle their students' natural curiosity about the "lifeworlds" of patients and their problems? From the students' own experiences most can undoubtedly recall encounters with pain, suffering, death, disability, joy, hope and despair, and the associated problems, complaints, conditions and symptoms—the language of disease—they engender. Most of the latter are readily understood on the basis of a sensitive conversation with the patient and often, as well, with the family or friends. Without such information is it possible for the physicians to construct a realistic history? A few more problems are clarified by closer observation of behavior and physical findings. At Wickenburg, Thomas Inui reported from his diary of patients cared for that 90 percent of them are in these first two categories. Only a tiny fraction require exposure to the full panoply of contemporary tertiary medical services. Is the task of medicine to be restricted to coping only with the tip of the iceberg while ignoring the rest (White, Williams, and Greenberg 1961)? If not, why then the disproportionate emphasis on the former while ignoring the latter?

Dr. Odegaard has recounted the sad history of medicine's

gradual drift from the liberating influence of the humanities and the study of man and his works. Another historian's recent account, *Bedside Manners: The Troubled History of Doctors and Patients*, is also essential reading for all who seek to understand the profession's current predicament (Shorter 1985). Shorter traces the history of doctor–patient relationships and their evolving attitudes, expectations and interactions from the eighteenth century to our present sorry state. Two centuries ago the profession was composed of "traditional" doctors, characterized by their authoritarian demeanor as purveyors of drugs, most of dubious benefit who, at the same time, were revered for their "healing powers," i.e., the placebo and Hawthorne effects and Factor X. On the other hand, the "traditional" patients of the day had their attachments to home remedies, accompanied by a strange combination of innate skepticism and unquestioning faith in doctors. From these origins and the beginning of scientific medicine, Shorter traces the patient–physician relationship to what he calls the postmodern era. Although more skilled and knowledgeable about the biological aspects of disease, today's doctors are seen to have focused on diseases to the neglect of the patients who have those diseases and have ignored the psychological and social components of those diseases. Concurrently there has been an increase in knowledge and accompanying anxiety about illness on the part of the public, which has increased the demand for understanding and explanation. A combination of technological wizardry and massive failure to understand the psychological and social origins and impacts of illness reflects multiple failures at the individual patient–physician level. The present impasse at a societal level as reflected in the popular press is the result (Blundell 1987; Eastabrook 1987).

Many additional reasons for this unhappy state of affairs were identified in the papers and discussions at Wickenburg, including: restriction of the venue for medical education to tertiary care teaching hospitals; selection bias with respect to both faculty and students; assignment of top priority in clinical teaching to diagnosis rather than to prognosis and resolution and management of patients' problems; lack of a clear understanding of the diagnostic process in either its probabilistic, or even its deterministic, modalities and resultant lack of useful frameworks for learning it; the notion that disease is fully understood and explained in terms of biological deviations; inability of faculty and residents to tolerate uncertainty and ambiguity; the monoetiological notion of causality in medicine (in contrast to the multifactorial assumptions used in other scientific undertakings directed at understanding, for example, the weather, earthquakes, ocean currents, bird migration, herd behavior and such service endeavors as management of airline capacity, just-in-time inventory control and even manipulation of financial markets); preoccupation with applying what is technologically feasible to the neglect of trying to understand what is not known; failure to read and appreciate all that Abraham Flexner wrote and meant; and, finally, use of a narrow mechanistic model of disease—based on the automotive culture in which so many American physicians and their patients seem to live.

Thorough reviews and clear expositions of some of these and related issues bearing on our knowledge about caring in relationship to the technological process are to be found in the paper discussed by Dennis Novack (1987) at Wickenburg and in recent volumes by two eminent physicians and clinical teachers, Mack Lipkin (1987) and Eric Cassell (1985). All three authors have reviewed the extensive clinical evidence bearing on the essential requirement that every physician should develop to a high degree skills in physician-patient communications, especially through interviewing. These skills are not "picked up" as the student or resident moves along, nor are they part of some nebulous "art" of medicine characterized as the "touchy-feely" school; they can be explicitly taught and learned. Well-known (in some circles) and extensively tested methods exist for eliciting and validating oral and behavioral interactions and communications.

At the Conference Douglas Drossman (1987), Thomas Inui (Inui, Yourtee, and Williamson 1976), Mack Lipkin, Jr. (Lipkin, Quill, and Napodano 1984), and Robert Smith (1986) demonstrated and discussed these skills. This new generation of young faculty members, supported by many of their senior colleagues, argued that acquisition of interviewing and communications skills is not only a desirable means, but probably the only means, for both appreciating and applying a more inclusive model of health and disease. Interviewing, as a means of history taking, is the single most important skill for enhancing the capacities of physicians and other medical personnel to understand and to help their patients while defining ever more precisely the task of medicine. The widespread disregard of inteviewing as an essential clinical skill to be learned in the course of a medical education may be a major reason for the public's current dissatisfaction with the profession.

The medical profession should not confuse its own views about patients and their ills with the views of the patients themselves and the public. The latter too have strong opinions about physicians and their works. Creative tensions between the medical profession and society are not new; the social contract governing what amounts to the "apostolic succession" that endows physicians with their powers and perquisites is under continuous renegotiation. In the final analysis society always determines the values and standards and the content of its contracts with the medical profession. Jay Katz puts the issue clearly in *The Silent World of Doctor and Patient*:

> It is dangerous nonsense to assert that in the practice of their art and science physicians can rely on their benevolent intentions, their abilities to judge what is the right thing to do, or their capacities for conducting their rounds with humanity, patience, prudence, and wisdom—all supposedly acquired through on-the-job training. It is not that easy. Medicine is a complex profession and the interactions between physicians and patients are also complex . . .
>
> What is true for physicians is equally true for patients. They, too, must learn that it is in their best interests to appreciate better than they now do that the practice of medicine is to a great extent still shrouded in uncertainty and that its practitioners, however competent and dedicated, are also fallible human beings. (Katz 1984)

Why do so many segments of the profession persist in ignoring patients' colloquial expressions of their health problems? What do people mean when they say: Don't do that to me or I'll have a stroke!; He died of a broken heart!; I was so terrified I almost had heart failure!; She was so discouraged she gave up!; and so on? Is this just so much babble? Suppose that it is. Surely the patient's concept of the genesis of his or her distress, as well as the patient's description of its effects on function and outlook, must have something to do with the prospects for understanding and resolving the problem constructively. Not so, if the seventeenth century model or automotive models are in vogue, but very much so, if a more inclusive twentieth century model is invoked.

The power of cultural factors to influence both the patient's and the physician's perception of the problems and what to do about them is illuminated by cross-national comparisons. French, German, English and American medical care for like problems is compared qualitatively and quantitatively by Lynn Payer, a medical journalist, in a forthcoming volume (Payer 1988). No matter what the language of discourse, similar complaints or symptom complexes—some far from trivial—are attributed to different "causes," given different labels, different remedies and different prognoses in the several countries considered. The overall health status of the populations, as measured by currently available methods, in all four countries is similar!

The role of traditional medicine in the developing world is well recognized. In China, separate medical schools including one of the five national "key" (i.e., elite) schools, train large numbers of traditional practitioners who apparently fill a societal need. In the Western world nonmedical health practitioners of various persuasions also seem to be meeting at least some of the perceived needs of a growing proportion of the public. To the extent that the medical profession, particularly in the face of a predicted surplus of physicians in the United States and Canada, does not respond to the public's expressed needs, we must surely be regarded as failing. If we do not wish to invoke the criteria of the marketplace, then we should strive to fulfill our collective professional responsibility for meeting the public's demands and expectations by defining our task for all to know and debate. At the most extreme, to put it bluntly, "there must be something wrong with patients who visit doctors when there is nothing 'wrong' with them!"

In other service endeavors the customer is usually deemed to be right until there is clear evidence to the contrary; not so in medicine. Why is it necessary for the *Wall Street Journal*, the *New York Times*, the *Washington Post* and *Newsweek*, to mention some of the more prominent print media, to run extensive articles and even supplements, not just "Op-Ed" pieces, describing the serious problems besetting doctor-patient communications in America? There appears to be widespread and growing concern that somehow and in some fashion the medical profession has a distorted view both of its task and of the health problems besetting society.

Why does *Love, Medicine & Miracles: Lessons Learned About Self-Healing from a Surgeon's Exceptional Patients* become a national best seller (Siegel 1987)? Some innate yearning must exist for deeper appreciation of the patient's "lifeworld" in which the disease arose and to which the patient returns after encounters with the medical establishment. This yearning seems to be increasingly accompanied by greater "learning" on the part of the public and their patients about the multiple factors that influence health and disease. We as a profession should strive to understand this yearning at the individual and collective levels, as we define the task of medicine. We should strive to understand our patients' problems in their terms; we should confine our interventions to those of demonstrated efficacy; we should use our own therapeutic powers (Factor X) at every opportunity; we should explain the limits of what we know and don't know; and we should state clearly where more research is needed.

The range of socioeconomic, cultural and ethnic backgrounds of medical students has broadened in the past decade or two. This is a desirable shift but much more is required to provide all students with an adequate appreciation of the even greater range of experiences, values, preferences, traditions and standards of the patients they will encounter. Without an adequate intellectual basis on which to develop their capacities for linguistic and semantic understanding and for empathy, it is hard to see how medical students can respond appropriately to patients' whose religious and cultural backgrounds, whose colloquial expressions, thresholds for expressing pain and disability and for seeking help differ greatly from those of the students and the physicians themselves. In the course of considering all these issues the student needs an opportunity to better understand her or his own origins, beliefs, values, attitudes and even conflicts and inhibitions. "Physician know and heal thyself!" is still a worthwhile dictum.

During the thirty years since Gartly Jaco (1958) published his anthology, a substantial body of new anthropological and sociological research has accumulated. Excellent volumes suitable for medical students abound; the introduction to a recent collection of research reports—*The Anthropology of Medicine: From Culture to Method*—describes the problem succinctly:

> Whatever else the diagnosis may be, it is first a social process based on interpersonal communication between the scientifically knowledgeable physician and the concerned patient. The physician should understand why and when a person seeks medical attention, how he [sic] views his own sickness, how he reports his symptoms and interprets his feelings, and what changes in his life occur because of his illness or treatment. These factors are always influenced by the respective cultural backgrounds of patient and physician. Wide variation in patients' backgrounds and the cultural differences between doctor and patient may profoundly influence the diagnostic process and therapeutic course. (Romanucci-Ross, Moerman, and Trancredi 1983)

Diagnosing and labeling seem to be the names of the contemporary medical exercises played most of the time by most of our medical students and house staff in most of our teaching hospitals. "You don't have 'it' until we name 'it' and when we do you have 'it'!" Several points warrant emphasis in discussing the code words doctors use to describe the phenomena with which they deal. The first is that nosography has a long and instructive history recounted in Faber's definitive volume (Faber 1930); this little classic should be read by every academic clinician for an informed perspective on the use of medical language and diagnostic fashions. Over the centuries both nomenclatures and classifications of human ills have changed in the light of the underlying concepts of causation. There is no reason to believe that they will not change in the future. Moreover they vary from culture to culture and often within cultures. Labels or diagnoses are the abstract code words doctors use as shorthand for the selected aspects of their patients' underlying phenomena they choose to observe and emphasize.

The International Classification of Diseases (ICD) has grown in response to clinical pressure groups with diverse notions about both the underlying concepts of causation and what to do about them. The ICD too has a long history, which is selectively recounted in the Introduction of its Ninth Revision (ICD 1977). The contemporary result is a bizarre and unwieldy mixture of chapters based on selected concepts of etiology, morphology, organ systems, clinical specialties, sex, age groups and treatment modalities. In attempting to satisfy so many special interest groups, such as clinical subspecialties, the evolutionary process that has characterized the development of the ICD seems to satisfy few. Advances in molecular biology, immunology and genetics are not adequately reflected and many clinical, especially primary care, needs are neglected. The ICD is based on an obsolete and unrealistic scheme; the time is ripe for rethinking and restructuring it (Feinstein 1987; White 1985).

We have known for thirty years that some 60 percent of problems presenting to a primary care physician cannot be assigned a suitable rubric from the *International Classification of Diseases* (College of General Practitioners 1958). So what do we do? We force what are really symptoms, problems, complaints or conditions into states which may or may not ensue and label them "diseases." And worse; we count them in our health statistics as if the "diseases" actually existed. But "if you can't label it, you can't count it; if you can't count it, it doesn't exist and, therefore, is not worth labeling!" This Catch-22 problem has plagued medicine and its health statistics over the centuries and warrants much more attention than it has received to date.

To compound the labeling problem further, the United States government in its infinite wisdom pays for hospital care, and perhaps soon ambulatory care, through a system that forces all problems into an ever more reified set of some 467 Diagnosis Related Groups (DRGs) (Office of Technology Assessment 1983) with little respect for accompanying social pathology or functional status. This system not only defies clinical experience but is statistically weak (Manton and Vertrees 1984). Patients do not come in "average" packages, they tend to be more or less like the extremes of some range or more precisely a vector of several ranges including, for example, functional status, severity, urgency, rate of change of the disease and therapeutic processes. There are many factors apart from the biological that affect where an individual patient fits on some continuum. Those concerned with the twentieth century model of health and disease, and even many physicians in clinical practice, find the notion of DRGs a mind-boggling distortion of reality.

Once more, we have known for about thirty years that social and psychological factors are more useful for prognosis than biological factors (Querido 1959 and 1963). Yet, the major preoccupation of the American academic medical establishment seems to be with manipulating the DRG system so that revenues are increased, rather than in thinking through the fundamental problem it seeks to address. More attention should be paid to the root causes of our present predicament.

Relief is in sight! A Working Party initially established by the World Health Organization (WHO) and carried forward by the World Organization of National Colleges, Academies, and Academic Associations of General Practitioners/Family Physicians (WONCA), has developed, after three major iterations, extensive international field evaluation, and tests of validity and reliability (far more rigorous than anything previously attempted for the ICD), the International Classification of Primary Care (ICPC) (Lamberts and Wood 1987); this volume is truly an innovation. More than a classification for the problems encountered in primary care, the ICPC provides a matrix of seven component modules for recording the natural progression of clinical understanding and management from initial presenting problems, symptoms, conditions and complaints through investigations, diagnoses, treatments, other interventions and administrative procedures. Each of the components is arrayed across thirteen chapters for bodily systems, including one each for female and male genital problems, a chapter for pregnancy, childbearing and family planning, two chapters for psychological and social problems and one for general conditions. The major conceptual breakthrough exemplified by the ICPC should not only guide the restructuring of future revisions of the ICD, and a family of related classifications, but it should facilitate the study of health and disease using expanded and more inclusive concepts and theories than those constrained by the present outmoded ICD.

This new classification also has been field-tested by WHO, supported by the U.S. National Institute of Mental Health, in primary care settings as a Triaxial Classification. After each patient encounter with a physician an entry is made on each of three axes, i.e., for the biological, psychological and social components of the patient's problem. This format focuses, and even demands, the clinician's attention to each of the three dimensions of the encounter and should encourage more accurate elicitation of clinical information, especially psychological and social information, and also more responsive interventions (Lipkin and Kupka 1982).

The second point is that for an unknown, but probably substantial, number of patients and their problems apparently we now have a set of labels which betokens ignorance of the underlying problems, overt hostility towards the patients, inability to tolerate uncertainty and ambiguity and fear about incapacity to help. What on earth has happened to a helping, caring, and even science-based, profession that refers to some of its patients (or since we apparently now seek to increase our market share, its "customers") in such dehumanizing terms as "crocks," "trolls," "gomers" (Get Out of My Emergency Room), "grunts," "dirtballs," "dirtbags," "drooling cretins," "squirrel bait" ("nuts"), "tobashs" (Take Out Back and Shoot in the Head) and much more (Cohen-Cole 1983, Donnelly 1986, and Easterbrook 1987).

Use of pejorative and demeaning clinical jargon to label those patients with difficult, misunderstood or chronic problems implies that an antiscientific mind-set has taken the place of humility, awe, curiosity and the accompanying motivation required to understand and to help. Use of dehumanizing and denigrating

43

labels represent a primitive defensive response to the open-ended, complex and often insoluble problems residents and physicians face, especially in tertiary care settings. "Problems that have solutions are not problems!" John Updike reminds us.

The absence of appropriate formal nomenclatures and classifications for 60 percent of our patients' health problems compounds matters. This pervasive neglect of adequate terms to describe patients' personal suffering, disability and feelings has contributed substantially to our present turmoil. Failure to develop and adopt realistic labels to describe our patients' suffering and the substitution of pejorative ones constitutes a *medical scandal*.

One response to all this has been *A Guide to Awareness and Evaluation of Humanistic Qualities in the Internist* promulgated by the American Board of Internal Medicine (1985). Again, this is a laudable exercise in remedial training, like teaching yuppie investment bankers table manners, but does anyone seriously believe that young physicians who have completed their residency training will fundamentally change their language and their attitudes just to surmount the hurdles of certification? Perhaps so, but certainly rigorous evaluation will be required to make the point. Although many of the problems are attitudinal and behavioral and have much to do with the selection of candidates for medical school, many others are structural and will require institutional changes that reflect a much broader concept of the task of medicine than seems to prevail today.

Prompt steps should be taken by deans, department heads, hospital administrators and others who aspire to being leaders to stop the use of such dehumanizing language. The word should go forth that this language and its implied behavior will no longer be tolerated. As Dody Bienenstock pointed out at Wickenburg, an essential ingredient in bringing about changes of this type is the sending of an unequivocal message from the senior faculty members and administration with respect to the attitudes and behavior that students and residents should exhibit towards patients; demeaning, dehumanizing and hostile behavior is unacceptable and will result in dismissal. Equally important will be the efforts taken to understand the root causes of this behavior and help students and residents to cope and to care.

The changes that are engulfing us scientifically, politically and economically behooves serious consideration of our collective task by using a bottom-up or population-based approach to appreciating and even understanding the genesis of society's health problems as individuals experience and describe them. The resultant restructuring of our medical schools and our health care arrangements from the bottom up will not come easily, but if the profession itself, especially its academic leaders, does not undertake this responsibility then, in the United States, it will most likely be undertaken by health care corporations organized under the auspices of diverse groups: investor-owned entities, insurance conglomerates, labor unions, doctors, hospitals, consumers' groups, municipalities, political jurisdictions and others.

Tragically, the ubiquitous domination of the medical establishment's thought and action by the seventeenth century model constrains the search for new kinds of evidence that might well bring new explanations and innovative interventions, to add to those based on that model. Of more mundane and immediate concern to politicians, this limited perspective is helping to push our health care establishment ever closer to bankruptcy. Resorting to increasingly expensive hospital-based technological interventions and a form of clinical reasoning that places high value on "not missing" or "ruling out" disorders of low probability is substituted for continuing management by science-based primary care physicians who focus on their patients' "lifeworlds" and the early, ambulatory care of them and their problems. The object of this fundamental service is to keep people functioning in their natural habitats and out of hospitals—necessary as the latter are at times. All this betokens a substantial down-sizing of the whole hospital industry in America accompanied by major increases in the primary care sector and restructuring of health care systems to link the three levels of care into effective systems. Integrated airlines and oil companies do this all the time; the medical establishment now faces the need to do the same in the

45

face of the reality of the population's needs, demands and willingness to pay, or, as some prefer, the pressures of the "market place."

There is enormous good will, boundless talent and extraordinary dedication within the greater medical profession. To effect change, however, we need to be clear about the impediments that face us; they are numerous and formidable.

IMPEDIMENTS TO CHANGE

OUR ACADEMIC COLLEAGUE, Dr. Odegaard, a layman, a friend of the medical profession, and a distinguished scholar, has defined our problem in its broadest dimensions in *Dear Doctor*. The other papers presented at the Conference served to illustrate and strengthen his message that now, more than ever in living memory, change is essential; and now is the time to start. In spite of its wondrous contributions to curative and even preventive medicine the present narrowly defined seventeenth century model seems to leave large components of the submerged part of the iceberg of pain, suffering, disability and disease untouched, mislabeled and often regarded as intractable (Last 1963). This outmoded model seems unable to accommodate much of the available historical, scientific and clinical evidence pointing to the major contributions made to the genesis of disease by social and psychological factors.

Dr. Odegaard has been careful to avoid a confrontational stance. As befits an historian he has examined and arrayed the evidence, including his own extensive experiences with the medical establishment and with medical education and its institutions. As such, his views should carry more weight, perhaps, than those of many medical proponents of the broader twentieth century model. Although the limitations of the biomedical model have been reviewed and the deficiencies and biases of modern American academic medicine emphasized, the advocates of the more inclusive model have clearly failed to convince the greater medical establishment of its merits and applicability. Shifts in thinking that have characterized theoretical physics and changed values and perspectives stemming from the work of philosophers of science have been noted earlier; apart from our

47

watershed advances in molecular biology, neurosciences, immunology and genetics, we have made little progress in addressing other equally transcendental matters.

What is to be lost by embracing a more inclusive model for understanding health and disease since no one suggests that the advances wrought through biomedical developments should be curtailed? The Wickenburg conferees seemed to agree that recognition of the need for change has to be supplemented by an overall strategy for accomplishing it both now and in the future.

Much of the evidence advanced in support of the viability of the broader model has been anecdotal and descriptive. Although valuable, such evidence scarcely provides an adequate basis for establishing a widely accepted new paradigm, especially one that appears to be as threatening to some as the biopsychosocial model. Collection of a dozen or even a thousand instances of loosely defined intrafamilial strife or occupational stress linked to subsequent ill health categorized by the rubrics of the *International Classification of Diseases* is not sufficient to establish the importance of psychological and social, in addition to biological, influences on specific medical ailments.

Nor, intriguing and important as the pioneering work of Ader, Richter and others has been, is it sufficient to use biological changes in small animals in response to environmental changes as a basis for extrapolating to human disease. Decreases in the use of health services accompanying patient-physician encounters characterized by the patient talking and the physician listening do not make the case for a broader model either. They all help and certainly none of them detract but it is going to take much more in the way of systematic investigation on a large scale to test the broad applicability of the twentieth century model. Just as traditional basic and clinical biomedical research is littered with flawed studies (Bailar and Mosteller 1986) so are contributions from the proponents of the more inclusive theory.

There is an urgent need to undertake carefully designed analytical and experimental studies that include collaboration among scientists working in wet laboratories, in hospitals and clinics and in populations. It is unlikely that much of this new brand of research can be done solely on patients attending tertiary care medical centers or by investigators isolated intellectually and institutionally from one another. Prospective, coordinated studies are needed that involve primary care physicians, epidemiologists, anthropologists, sociologists, experimental psychologists, immunologists, geneticists, molecular biologists and pharmacologists. The potential benefits from problem-based collaborative laboratory, clinical and social investigations is well illustrated by the recent genetic, laboratory and population studies of Janice Egeland and her colleagues on bipolar disease (Egeland et al. 1987).

The predictive nature of the experiments and the generalizability of the results are what give credence and bring acceptance to the underlying theories—until the next new paradigm emerges. To date this kind of large-scale original analytical and experimental research has been in short supply. With a few notable exceptions, it is not seen as important by government and philanthropic funding agencies, by the academic establishment, by journal editors or, apart from a hardy band of truly creative fundamental neuroscientists and behavioral scientists, by the armies of orthodox clinical investigators plodding along under the banner of the received wisdom of the day—the seventeenth century model.

The short answer is that many of the people with creative research questions do not seem to know much about sound research methods. And conversely, many of those with a knowledge of sound methods of inquiry seem to lack both the spark of creative curiosity and direct exposure to the problems that should inspire them to ask important questions. There is an urgent need for promising young investigators to receive thorough training in the design, measurement and evaluation methods required to test hypotheses bearing on the more inclusive model of health and disease. There is an equally urgent need to stimulate young investigators to ask creative questions derived, if not from the "lifeworlds" of their patients, then from a broader exposure to the human condition through biography, history and fiction.

Compared to the biological factors, the intense investigation of which has yielded such extraordinary benefits for mankind, the psychological and social parameters are too often seen by many young academicians as barren territory for research, just as they are in the care of patients. With the biomedical model successfully bolstered by the dualism of Descartes, the reductionism of Newton and the automotive culture of General Motors, change is held to be unnecessary by most and impossible by a few. As George Engle put it, we are faced with "the notion of the body as a machine, of disease as a consequence of breakdown of the machine, and the doctor's task as repair of the machine" (Engle 1977).

Alan Gregg is alleged to have said that the two worst mistakes made by the Rockefeller Foundation were to support Departments of Psychiatry in American medical schools in which psychoanalysis was the *sole* "basic" science and to create separate schools of public health apart from medical schools. At the time both decisions were seen as appropriate initiatives to broaden medicine's concerns for the influence on health and disease, of psychological factors, on the one hand, and of environmental and population-based factors, on the other. Apart from their unquestionably constructive imports, both decisions have had far-reaching, and clearly unforeseen, negative perturbations for American medical research, education and practice.

The first decision was designed to bring the insights of Freud into the bastions of academic medicine, which after World War II was already energetically pursuing an ever-narrowing vision of the biomedical model reinforced by the limited reading of Flexner. Although research and teaching on interviewing was developing in nonmedical academic sectors, the advent of psychoanalytic teaching may have done more than anything else to develop and refine the skills of medical interviewing, especially the skills required to listen and observe. We learned much about patient-physician interactions and communications from the psychoanalysts and not a little about ourselves, as Robert Smith reminded us at Wickenburg (Smith 1986). But useful as the introduction of Freud's insights has been, sole dependence on psychoanalysis for underpinning psychiatric practice and for understanding many of the psychological complexities of medicine has had the unfortunate effect, until quite recently, of depriving psychiatry and all it stands for of a substantial experimental basic science. Again the issue is not solely one of quantification but there are issues of validity, reliability, generalizability and pre-dictability which have not been addressed by psychoanalysis to the satisfaction of even many of its supporters.

Much of the pioneering research and teaching by Maurice Levine, John Romano and George Engle and their colleagues, initiated at the Universities of Cincinnati and Rochester, and by Michael Balint in Britain, strove to overcome the institutional and conceptual barriers already enveloping medicine. But their views seem to have been given short shrift by the American medical establishment for almost forty years. The Rockefeller initiative in the 1950s took psychiatry out of the mainstream of the American version of scientific thought as medicine in its ef-forts to understand the human condition was increasingly re-stricting its vision to biological phenomena. There was, until quite recently, no basic science in the medical school concerned with psychological aspects of health and disease and hence no countervailing voice from an experimental science in the coun-cils of those teaching in the preclinical years of medical school and employing the biomedical model.

Today the neurosciences are filling part of that void. Some would argue, however, that even their clinical counterpart, bio-logical psychiatry, may be embracing the biomedical model too vigorously at the cost of ignoring nonbiological factors in the genesis of psychological disorders and mental illness—yet an-other instance of a narrow, instead of a broader, balanced, model guiding the task of medicine. We were told at Wickenburg that a recent survey of 1000 internal medicine residents determined that the total length of their exposure to any teaching about "mental health" (and it is not too clear what that means) was 45 minutes!

George Engel and his students and followers were, neverthe-less, much in evidence at Wickenburg and indeed their work generated most of the clinical, as distinguished from the histori-cal, background for the Conference. Their skills in investigating and teaching interviewing techniques demonstrated clearly at Wickenburg that the patient-physician relationship is central to the practice of scientific medicine and that the scientific examination of this relationship is central to defining medicine's individual and collective tasks. Gayle Stephens captured the importance of this relationship when he said, "The spoken word is the royal road to understanding in medicine!" For these insights, psychoanalysis, in spite of its limitations, gets much of the credit.

In a similar fashion, the population-based sciences, including epidemiology, demography, anthropology, sociology, economics and health statistics, with their extensive quantitative and interviewing skills, were, for the most part, relegated to schools of public health separated geographically, intellectually and conceptually from medical schools. As a consequence of this decision by the Rockefeller Foundation at the time of World War I, the faculties of these new schools have had little or no impact on mainstream scientific medicine and the paradigms that guided research, education and practice. Absent from the medical schools were the quantitative skills needed for critical appraisal of the medical literature and the avalanche of new maneuvers stemming from advances in biomedicine. Also absent was the population-based, epidemiological information essential for developing educational and research priorities and for guiding the organization of services. Nor did the public health faculties, in turn, benefit from rubbing shoulders with clinicians, patients and above all teachers and investigators in the medical schools.

The exclusion of psychiatry, experimental psychology, the behavioral sciences and population-based health disciplines from the heart of the medical establishment was in stark contrast to the integration of physics, chemistry and biology into the fabric of medical research and education in the Flexnerian era. These two major "mistakes" by the Rockefeller Foundation relegated psychological and social factors and their attendant scientific underpinnings as well as their humanizing influence, to increasingly isolated, and frequently denigrated, departments of psychiatry and schools of public health. Both were virtually barred from central roles in the evolution of modern medicine, its theories, practices and educational priorities. Those concerned with the impact of behavioral and environmental factors on health and disease worked in different arenas; and perhaps they attracted different types of faculty members and students. Their influence over the decades, with a few notable exceptions, has been modest, indeed, compared to that of the other "fundamental" medical scientists employing the natural sciences and the biomedical model.

There is an urgent need to examine the organizational and structural arrangements that keep those knowledgeable about the impact of psychological and social factors on health and disease out of critical decision-making processes in medical education and research and unable to influence the greater medical establishment's delineation of its task.

A rationally balanced set of health care arrangements should have its resources sized in relation to the distribution of the medical problems encountered by the population served. Common problems are common and rare problems are rare! In the United States the overall system is grossly out of balance. The ratios of tertiary care beds and of many subspecialists to ambulatory care facilities and to general physicians are reversed from those in most other industrialized countries. *Appropriately trained* primary care physicians are in short supply in the United States. No European countries, and certainly not Canada, Australia or New Zealand, have neglected their basic primary care services to the extent the United States has done since World War II. So highly regarded is primary medical care in Finland that general or family physicians must undergo *five years* of postgraduate training— the same as most specialists—before qualifying. The scope of competence is the important point, not the duration of training.

We now have a substantial part of almost two generations of leaders in American academic medicine who simply do not understand what primary care is all about. What is worse, far too many members of the contemporary medical establishment, in both basic and clinical departments, do not seem to appreciate the challenges and opportunities for research in primary care (Mair 1975; White 1976). Nor do they seem to appreciate the need to understand or provide services for those with "early," "trivial," "amorphous," "self-limited," "functional," "incurable," "intractable" or "chronic" disorders. Although these

conditions may not respond to contemporary tertiary care interventions, and have not stimulated much in the way of research
by academicians working in such settings, they involve untold
billions of days of suffering, dysfunction and work-loss and de-
vour huge amounts of money—money that might better be
spent on further fundamental research of all types into the
origins of such conditions and on further education designed to
improve their management.

Countries such as Finland, Norway, Sweden and the Netherlands and health maintenance organizations such as Kaiser Per-
manente seem to be able to size their resources and manpower
appropriately to meet the needs of the populations they serve.
Why not other health care enterprises? The most obvious reason
is that although the problems, issues and strategies for responding were all set out in Lord Dawson's Report of 1920 (Dawson
1920), most leaders of our contemporary medical establishment
have never heard of that Report and few have even thought
about the problems from a population perspective. In that seminal analysis of health care organization, Dawson and his colleagues set out the rationale for having three tiers of health services: primary, secondary and tertiary, and made specific
recommendations for the organization, staffing and responsibil-
ities of each.

There are at least four institutional barriers to improving the
situation so that the full range of interrelated biological, social
and psychological health problems can be studied and the people
who experience them served.

First is the banishment of family medicine and, to a considerable extent, its ally and sister field, general internal medicine, to
minor roles with respect to curriculum time, real estate, patient
populations, professional status, pay and other trappings of academic power.

Second is the assumption that the present disarray is best improved by the formation of horizontal cartels of hospitals and
nursing homes, when vertically integrated systems are really
needed, which balance resources and manpower in relation to
needs (Dawson 1920; Engle 1968).

The third barrier is the constricted view of the full spectrum of health problems experienced by most medical faculties—a view that derives from their brief, often transient, exposure to highly selected patient populations (White, Williams, and Greenberg 1961). The majority of the clinical faculty have been exposed only to rare conditions, the "sickest" patients and the most complicated diseases. The care of the latter is absolutely necessary—no question about it—however, the exposure of the faculty is limited to but a small fraction of society's total medical and health problems, and even that exposure concentrates on biological factors to the exclusion of the social and psychological.

Fourth is the tendency of subspecialists of various persuasions to band together, seeming to have many characteristics of self-serving, national organizations closely allied with their bureaucratic colleagues and political patrons, to whom they often seem to owe greater allegiance than to their own universities, hospitals or health care systems, to say nothing of their patients and the populations their institutions serve.

These four institutional and professional constraints have produced structural limitations which collectively make change extremely difficult. The latest response from the medical establishment to this predicament is not reassuring (Task Force on Academic Health Centers 1985). The Task Force seems to have examined the whole health care apparatus from the viewpoint of the tertiary care teaching hospital, rather than from the viewpoints of the populations and their perceived needs, and now from the crescendo of expressed demands. The medical profession must be the only service or production enterprise extant that organizes itself top-down from the supply-side alone; every other service organization examines the needs and demands of its customers, or the demographics of the population served, and plans bottom-up from a "market," demographic or epidemiologic information base. This truly bizarre state of affairs is all the more astonishing since the problem was laid out almost seventy years ago in unusually lucid language by Lord Dawson (1920).

That "cognitive" medicine—another piece of jargon that tends to reify the listening and counseling ministrations of the medical profession ever more—is much less lucrative than "procedural" medicine is not news. Similarly, much hospital care is paid for more generously than ambulatory care. And finally, the prospective "reimbursement" system presently in vogue is based on the final diagnoses (DRGs) rather than on patients' presenting problems and their satisfactory management and resolution. With procedures, hospitals and diagnoses taking precedence for payment and resources within the narrow biomedical paradigm, how can those not at the center of the establishment expect to attract resources for prevention of disease and promotion of health, for caring and managing their patients' problems? How can social, familial and community resources that appear to be so efficacious in supporting and healing the sick be integrated and coordinated (Haggerty 1987 and Medalie 1976)? Nor is there the intellectual environment or incentive to conduct further research into the influence of support systems on the origins and course of disease and its related medical care, or to inquire into the comparative costs of different sites and modalities of care.

There is undoubtedly a substantial residue of altruism in medicine and it retains at least some of the ideals, if not the outward manifestations, of a learned profession, but the perverse financial incentives in which we are now enmeshed are extremely difficult to disregard, especially for students contemplating medicine as a career, for new medical graduates and even for many practitioners. As long as the pecuniary rewards in medicine ignore such elements as time devoted to listening, observing and explaining, experience and wisdom in dealing with interpersonal, domestic, occupational and social stress, simple ambulatory management based on "wait-and-see" as a diagnostic or therapeutic maneuver, and a probabilistic, rather than a deterministic, approach to dealing with the patient's problem, it seems unlikely that a more inclusive theory of health and disease will find widespread acceptance.

A massive educational effort will be required to convince the public and its politicians that the pecuniary, and surely the humanitarian, rewards from investigating the psychological and social, in addition to the genetic, nutritional, environmental and biological, influences on health and disease, especially at the level of primary care, are likely to equal or surpass those that have resulted from the more limited biomedical approach that now prevails.

Any medical school with one or two full-time faculty in its clinical departments skilled in talking with "run-of-the-mill," undifferentiated patients is indeed fortunate. If, in addition, these faculty members have a setting in which they can care for their patients throughout assorted manifestations of health and disease over a period of months or years, the situation must indeed be unusual. The old G.P. is not the model; it is rather the contemporary primary care physician with exemplary training based on the twentieth century model discussed at the Wickenburg Conference. Apart from the skills and sensitivity needed to listen, hear and observe, the ideal role model will have the requisite knowledge and skills to cope with at least 90 percent of the ills of her or his patients, and perhaps with another 5 percent or more after consultations from subspecialists.

Instead of seeking out these role models and providing the necessary institutional arrangements in which they can teach and conduct research, the current establishment simply urges more outpatient teaching, more often than not, based in its tertiary care teaching hospital. A few Family Medicine Teaching Centers and their faculty approach the desired model, but few of the faculty members control their own hospital beds in which they can care for their own patients, and fewer still care for a cross section of the population. General internists in academic medical centers frequently do not have their own inpatient hospital beds in which to care for their own ambulatory patients whom they admit. In neither instance can continuity of care be observed or learned and little is gleaned about the decisions to admit or discharge patients as they relate to prevention, early diagnosis, psychological and social support systems, home care, respite and palliative care. To make matters worse both family physicians and general internists in most academic settings are usually inundated with extremely heavy service loads required to earn their salaries. As Robert Haggerty pointed out at Wickenburg, it is ineffectual to attempt to teach medical students about "effective" care in environments that are clearly organizational and operational disasters. Medical students, like everyone else, learn

57

best in an environment where the teachers practice what they preach and provide first-rate, compassionate care that is science-based (behavioral, biological, and population-based sciences) and responds to the patient's perceived problems. At present most teaching hospitals are simply not organized to achieve this for either their students or their patients. You cannot do good teaching in a bad system!

Those medical centers with family medicine or general internal medicine faculty appropriately trained to conduct research within the broader model considered at Wickenburg, although still rare, are increasing in numbers and quality. The combined track records in research from both camps may leave much to be desired, but those representatives at Wickenburg gave reason for optimism. Their future contributions to understanding the biopsychosocial model, particularly at the primary care level, through analytical and experimental studies—in contrast to talking about the twentieth century model—should emulate those of their biomedical colleagues in quality and quantity.

Interest in worthy enterprises and new paradigms is not synonymous with advancing scientific and humanistic understanding of health and disease; science and scholarship are the fundamental coins of academic discourse. Physicians who can apply the twentieth century model both in providing exemplary care and conducting first-rate research, as well as in teaching, require encouragement and nurturing. For research, especially, the faculty member needs protected time to reflect and plan worthwhile studies. Is it any wonder that progress has been slow without adequate administrative and financial support from deans, department heads, and funding agencies? But in addition, those who seek to undertake clinical research in departments of family medicine and divisions of general internal medicine and general pediatrics require suitable training to the point where they are independent investigators. Without this they are likely to continue reinventing the wheel and their contributions are likely to be modest. Again Alvan Feinstein states the case clearly:

> The interventional activities of patient care have always offered and continue to offer basic scientific challenges in the stimulating, creative, investigative use of clinical knowledge and skills. To allow modern medical

technology to be managed with both humanistic perception and scientific effectiveness, the basic strategies must come from a clinical scholarship that is rooted in the care of patients, aimed at the care of patients, and based on data and models that reflect the pertinent observations, events and care. The scholarship should be broad, wide-ranging, and receptive enough to include and apply the many valuable contributions that can come from other basic domains. The main intellectual challenge for clinicians today, however, is to develop the basic scientific models for which clinicians are the primary scholars and investigators. (Feinstein 1987)

In addition to all these circumstances, many current role models in academic medicine, especially in the subspecialties of internal medicine, are said to have only limited interactions with the patients for whom they are nominally responsible and who are fundamental to the educational process on the wards. It is rare, indeed, to have a live patient presented at grand rounds and rarer still to allow the patient to tell the story of the illness in his or her own words. One participant at the Wickenburg Conference stated that a survey of students elicited the startling finding that the attending physicians actually visited at the bedside and talked to patients only 20 to 30 percent of the time!

If the actual figure turns out to be even double this on a national scale it is devastating news—indeed a *second medical scandal*. Because of the temporal and spatial constraints of the tertiary care hospital, there is said to be minimal opportunity to appreciate and study the psychological and social aspects of disease and hence the necessity of limiting attention to the biological. Thomas Inui clearly demonstrated at Wickenburg that this state of affairs does not have to be accepted; bedside conversations and examinations that are sensitive and informative can be conducted by motivated and competent attending physicians. Without the essential skills, experience, knowledge and ensuing stimulation, is it little wonder that enquiry has been stifled and teaching has often been perfunctory? Without a reversal of this state of affairs, the prospects are grim indeed for broadening the model to consider the circumstances under which the patient's illness arose and to which he or she must return after a brief sojourn in the hospital.

An important initiative canvassed at Wickenburg (and also in other settings) started with the observation that since their numbers are so few and the problems so daunting would it not make sense for the family physicians and general internists to join forces? If they really believe that the available evidence supports the need for structured investigation and more effective teaching, as well as for exemplary patient care, using the twentieth century model, should they not abandon such ephemeral concerns as turf, status and their separate origins and traditions and merge? Perhaps, as several suggested in the informal talks during the Conference, they should preempt the term "physician" and become the "personal doctors" about which Sir Robert Fox, the distinguished editor of the *Lancet*, wrote so lucidly almost thirty years ago (Fox 1960). There must be common cores of knowledge, skills and concerns about which these two clinical fields could organize at least some, and eventually all, aspects of their teaching, patient care and research.

And what of the medical curriculum itself? One reason both preclinical and clinical medical textbooks have been so large is that there are so few general principles. Everything is recounted in enormous descriptive detail with the expectation that it can be recalled on demand. Contemporary learning and information theories and computer processing of information, as well as the advances in molecular biology, immunology and genetics, are changing all that. Under the present arrangements most medical students are exhausted by their intensive immersion in the several basic sciences, the application of which to clinical problems too often eludes them. Again the sciences "basic" to medicine are said to be the natural sciences. Psychology, sociology, anthropology, demography, epidemiology, economics and health statistics (as distinguished from biostatistics) too often are given cursory attention and generally denigrated by implication if not explicitly.

At the clinical level most students' exposure is restricted to desperately ill patients, unusual complications and rare diseases where the priorities are based on heroic, life-sustaining measures and on mastering some aspects of the diagnostic process. Although useful to a degree, these experiences are said to dull both awareness and interest in the many other facets of understanding and managing illness and disease. Once more, the problem is a matter of balance. There seems to have been no rational basis for the way the contemporary curriculum has been allowed to grow. And worse—there seem to be few effective mechanisms for fundamental review and change. Like the organization of the hospital and health services generally it is a top-down, supply-side approach. The challenge is to help students to think about the problems they will face and to learn new approaches for obtaining information about the principles involved and about the substantive details of specific applications. If there is any merit to the problems addressed at Wickenburg, then, at the very least, the balance among the full range of sciences fundamental to medicine's task needs radical rethinking. I believe Flexner would agree! Certainly Dr. Odegaard would.

Several innovations come from Canada. First, a wide-ranging international symposium on *Health in the 80's and 90's and Its Impact on Health Sciences Education* was:

> . . . designed with the general objective of providing participants with an understanding of the factors that influence human health, the nature of health care, the economic and political factors that affect human health and health care, the impact of professional bodies and attitudes on health and health care, the types of evidence that are used in decision-making and their impact on health and health care, and moral and ethical issues. (Squires 1983)

Fundamental examinations of the task of university health sciences centers from a population or public perspective must be rare indeed; this may well have been a first. Those interested in considering these matters further should find the proceedings of interest.

Second, the University of Ottawa now makes broad decisions about the context of its curriculum from an inventory of the health problems experienced by the population being served. Survey data generated by the "customers" constitutes the principal guide for discussing the organization of the curriculum rather than the current research interests of individual faculty members (Rosser and Beaulieu 1984). Is this really an unreasonable approach? At any rate Ottawa's new departure has apparently generated considerable interest in other medical schools in Canada and the United States. A similar innovation comes from

McMaster University where priorities for education are based on the frequency of the problems in the population served, on the availability of efficacious interventions, on the need for palliative and supportive care, and on the suitability of the problems as sound educational prototypes from which to learn broad principles (Chong et al. 1987).

Another related initiative is also being undertaken by McMaster University through Task Force II of the Network of Community-Oriented Educational Institutions for Health Sciences, with headquarters in the Faculty of Medicine at the Rijksuniversiteit Limburg, Maastricht, The Netherlands. This Network, supported by the World Health Organization and the Rockefeller and other foundations, consists of about thirty schools around the world committed, at least on paper, to directing their institutional efforts at meeting the health needs of the populations they serve. Task Force II is developing methods by which young faculty members from medical schools in both the developing and developed worlds can assess the qualitative and quantitative aspects of the burden of illness experienced by the populations in which their medical schools reside. An international advisory committee assists the McMaster faculty in guiding the fellows' work during two sojourns at McMaster six months apart (Neufeld 1987).

Perhaps the most innovative proposal for defining the task of medicine comes from the Pan American Health Organization (1986). A remarkable document sets forth a logical framework for determining educational priorities based on the health problems of the community served. Although the framework emphasizes demographic, social and economic factors as well as biologic, in defining each medical school's mission, incorporation of psychological factors should not prove difficult. The overall approach is stated clearly in the document's two opening paragraphs:

> It is important for every medical school to understand its situation with respect to what society, as a whole, and the school's own community expects and requires of the institution and its graduates to understand this in terms of social development, on the one hand, and technological and scientific development, on the other. Understanding this situation is the

first step towards improving it, and the course of action a school must take might be guided by general social expectations and the scientific and technological capacities of the school's human resources.

> It is necessary for those directly concerned to carry out this situational analysis since no one from outside who is unfamiliar with the school can have either sufficient familiarity with the institution or a real understanding of all the determining factors and circumstances affecting its existence and development. (Pan American Health Organization 1986)

The point of these bottom-up or population-based approaches to defining the task of medicine is that they seek to respond to the perceived needs of people and to define more clearly what types of efficacious interventions can be effectively and efficiently provided, while further research is pursued on those problems for which understanding and management strategies are lacking.

Other changes are afoot. The McMaster faculty has pioneered new methods of medical education that seek to emphasize behavioral and population factors as much as the more traditional biological; they have not always been uniformly successful but the effort continues. As a health sciences faculty, not just a medical faculty, they have established new standards worldwide in the use of problem-based learning and community-oriented priority setting. Similarly, the University of Missouri in Kansas City has attracted considerable attention by developing a problem-based curriculum staffed by preceptors who work with their students, admitted directly from high school, throughout the years of medical education. Both these universities have contributed ideas that have encouraged the Harvard Medical School to initiate its trial of a "New Pathway" curriculum.

Change is possible but it seems to come from either the brand "new" schools which start with pencil and paper or from the great "old" schools which may take a giant leap forward every couple of generations. Problem-based learning (which also needs to be the object of evaluation) is really an extension of the case method of teaching introduced by Walter B. Cannon at Harvard two generations ago. The term itself immediately gives rise to questions about the nature of the problems to be addressed; use of the problem-based method provides no innate assurance that psychological and social factors will be examined as diligently as biological factors. The nature of the underlying model to be used in medical education becomes central to the whole enterprise. Innovations in pedagogical maneuvers are no substitute for intensive concern with both the content of the learning and the models that shape that learning. Exactly what kinds of information are needed to estimate the types and dimensions of the population's collective medical problems and what information is needed to understand each individual's illness, its origins, its course, its management and its prospects?

At the center of our educational practices is the seventeenth century model which tends to reify and mislabel "the patient," "the diagnosis," and "the treatment." Our primary concern appears to be with the radio receiver itself and not with the origins, melody and transmission of the music. Or our concerns are with the automobile and not with the driver, where she or he is going and why. To introduce a twentieth century model which pays at least as much attention to the music and the driver as to the radio receiver and the automobile is going to be a formidable task indeed. But is this attention not really essential for delineating medicine's task?

All the proponents of a broadened model for medicine, including the enthusiastic cohort of younger clinical academicians at Wickenburg, have survived both the contemporary medical student selection process and the rigors of the allegedly truncated education they received under the umbrella of the biomedical model. However, it is of more than passing interest that many of those present had been trained or influenced either by Dr. Engle, the originator of the twentieth century model, or by Sydney Kark, the originator and principal proponent of new methods for applying the expanded model through what he calls "community-oriented primary care" (Kark 1981 and Nutting 1987). Individuals can and do make a difference. Dr. Odegaard's *Dear Doctor* will make a difference.

No one suggests that there is one and only one "right" type of medical student required to embrace and implement the twentieth century model. But would it not be well to pay more attention to the composition of medical school classes? Do we really have adequate information about the personal characteristics and interests of different types of physicians, especially about those who would be primary care physicians? Are they different from those who are so successful with the complex techniques of instrumentation? If psychologists can identify individuals with the capacity for "spatial thinking" to train as air traffic controllers, and with the capacity for "lateral thinking" to train as design engineers, could we not enlist their help in identifying more specifically the balance of aptitudes and talents we seek in the mix of entering medical students? Are there individuals suited to become future general physicians with quite different talents from those who do well in wet laboratory research, in instrumental specialties or in population-based research? Each group has its place but each may also require quite different types of people. Medical school admissions committees should know what those differences are and strive for a more responsive balance than we seem to have today. Wickenburg participants noted that a number of major departments of internal medicine failed this year to fill all their house staff quotas. This stark reality should stimulate the leaders of these departments to examine the root causes of this historic mismatch between the expectations of the teachers and the taught.

The feminization of American medicine will undoubtedly make a difference. And what would happen if we selected a large proportion of the classes from those with undergraduate majors in the humanities and the social sciences? The facts are that the average acceptance rate for undergraduates with majors in the humanities is 50.3 percent (with highs of 58.1 percent in music and 55.8 percent in philosophy) and those in the social sciences is 42.3 percent (with highs of 53.0 percent in economics and 45.7 percent in both history and political science). The acceptance rate for those with majors in the natural sciences is 45.7 percent. The message for undergraduates is clear: "If you want to be admitted to medical school, major in music!" And those with backgrounds in the humanities and social sciences do just as well in medical school as those with natural science majors (Bruer and Warren 1981).

Is it not also incumbent on medical admissions committees to determine whether or not there is good evidence that the candidate possesses the essential qualities of integrity, respect and compassion? As defined by the American Board of Internal Medicine (1985), these qualities are straightforward:

> Integrity is the personal commitment to be honest and trustworthy in evaluating and demonstrating one's own skills and abilities.

> Respect is the personal commitment to honor others' choices and rights regarding themselves and their medical care.

> Compassion is an appreciation that suffering and illness engender special needs for comfort and help without evoking excessive needs for emotional involvement which could undermine professional responsibility for the patient.

The problems of assessing these are substantial and the record poor, as discussed at some length in the Institute of Medicine's study, *Medical Education and Societal Needs: A Planning Report for the Health Professions* (1983). Nevertheless to leave the assessment of these essential personal qualities until the resident is preparing to take Board examinations in, say, internal medicine seems outrageously late. Public awareness of this state of affairs would surely generate yet a *third medical scandal*. If these qualities can be assessed in the course of residencies as a prelude to sitting the American Board of Internal Medicine's examinations, the same could be accomplished during clinical clerkships—especially if the residents were asked to do the assessing and were monitored by the faculty. Until adequate methods are developed for assessment of personal qualities at the time of admission to medical school their assessment in medical school seems mandatory.

If such qualities are positively identified in successful candidates for medical school it should be unnecessary to provide remedial training later on. However, given the present parlous state of the profession's relations with the public it would seem just as important to dismiss students from medical school for failing to demonstrate these qualities as it is for failing to understand some aspect of bioscience.

There is one final obstacle to acceptance of the broader, more inclusive model. In spite of the colloquial observations and the growing awareness about the importance of emotional and social genesis of much ill health, many segments of the American public share a widely held belief that every problem has a solution, that every solution involves a pill, procedure or some other intervention or a service, and that every service has, to use another frightening piece of jargon, a "provider!" Such wondrous developments have come from the revolutions wrought by molecular biology and immunology that the public has become accustomed to an unending stream of efficacious interventions. They may well be right.

The ubiquitous biomedical model, with its traditions and its "miracles," further distracts us from broadening the base of inquiry and learning. Why not stay the course and forget about the underbrush of psychological and social influences on health and disease? Why bother to listen or talk to patients? What is needed is more cure and less care! What I do, how I behave, how I react, my parents, my family, my job, my friends have nothing to do with how I feel or how I function! I am a radio set without an orchestra or music and an automobile without a driver or a destination! In the face of this set of beliefs and attitudes, it will be no easy matter to change our concepts of health and disease, of man and his place in the scheme of things. The latter are metaphysical matters but the former are matters of education—information, knowledge and perhaps even wisdom.

We are back to where Dr. Odegaard in *Dear Doctor* started with his account of the tragic split between scientific and humanistic studies. We have inherited the narrow view of our potential scientific endeavors bequeathed us by an incredibly isolated American medical establishment during the last half century.

True, the medical establishment cannot take on the reformation of American society or its educational apparatus but it can do something about the education of its own and it can help the media to educate the public. In many ways, as suggested earlier in this essay, both the public and the media are showing increasing signs of restlessness and there is growing skepticism about the adequacy of present health care arrangements to cope at either the individual or collective levels.

Information is certainly one of the keys: information about the origins, nature and distribution of our patients, symptoms, complaints, impairments, disabilities, problems; information about the efficacy of available interventions; information about the therapeutic powers of family and community support systems, of the placebo and Hawthorne effects of Factor X, of the "relaxation response," of hope and of love; information about needed research of all types. We need information, and even more knowledge and wisdom about ourselves—as individuals and physicians. Above all, we need information from our patients about their "lifeworlds;" the stuff of clinical interviews but also the stuff of novels, biographies, poetry and art. *Dear Doctor* sets us on the right course—perhaps the course from biomedicine to infomedicine. "I like to think of myself," said Thomas Inui, possibly speaking for many at the Conference, "as a physician interested in all the ways of knowing."

NEXT STEPS

THE CONFERENCE REACHED no formal conclusions, passed no resolutions and made no specific recommendations. The object of the exercise was to start a national dialogue initiated by *Dear Doctor* and extended by the papers presented at Wickenburg and the discussions that took place. Informally, and inferentially during discussions, there were, however, many suggestions placed on the table. The following themes cover most of the feasible opportunities for exercising maximum leverage directed at broadening acceptance of the twentieth century model of health and disease. No one initiative is likely to result in prompt adoption of a more inclusive conceptual framework for investigating, teaching and practicing medicine; indeed that is not the objective. Together, however, they could produce shifts at the periphery so that both necessary, and eventually sufficient, fundamental change might occur. Although hard to detect at the time, in retrospect a "paradigm shift" might be seen to have occurred. At the least there is the hope that discussion of these "next steps" will enlarge and enhance the national dialogue.

I turn, therefore, to a discussion of eight broad initiatives that should serve to establish the facts about the facts and help us to define the task of medicine more clearly. The steps proposed are at once designed to restore leadership to a beleaguered academic medical establishment and above all to assure the American public that its concerns are heard. All the suggestions should be viewed as positive. None should in any way threaten those advancing our understanding of the biological components of disease so productively; perhaps they will be encouraged to join in expanding the perspectives from which they pursue their own contributions to the task of medicine.

INTERVIEWING AND COMMUNICATION SKILLS

The widespread lack of interviewing skills and the accompanying impediments to constructive communication with patients
appear to have been well-documented by the Society of General
Internal Medicine's (SGIM) Task Force on Interviewing and Related Skills. The best evidence for perceived deficiencies in these
skills is to be found in the enormous demand for attendance at
the faculty workshops the Task Force conducts and in the demand for teaching materials. This apparent deficiency in what
many believe to be a fundamental clinical skill for all physicians
who have any direct contacts with patients deserves national attention by the AAMC and its constituent medical schools.

One way to move matters further and faster is for the National
Board of Medical Examiners (NBME) to add a set of final examination problems or questions that make it clear to students
and faculty alike that competence in these skills is just as important as knowledge of the biosciences and of clinical interventions; all three sets of skills and knowledge are essential, and
although clinical skills other than interviewing and communication could be assessed, the suggestion here is that the initial
examination be limited to these latter two skills, using standardized patients (Stillman et al. 1986), one-way screens and standardized interview rating forms (Stillman et al. 1977 and Institute of Medicine 1983, p. 67, reference 21) or any other suitable
method. There are few matters that would reassure the public
more than to know that, together with a traditional medical education, their physicians have achieved competence in interviewing and communication. Specialty boards should introduce
similar standards and examinations.

In addition to the setting of standards by the NBME and the
specialty boards, there will need to be a quantum increase in the
faculty resources devoted to teaching these skills. So far has the
situation deteriorated that even the teachers of the teachers are in
scarce supply. Each medical school should have a critical mass of
physicians, composed of family physicians, general internists
and general pediatricians, augmented by psychiatrists, obstetri-
cians and general surgeons, and supported by behavioral scien-

tists, who provide dedicated training modules, including video-tapes, for other faculty and residents initially and then for medical students. There is little point in training the latter, if the former two groups do not provide appropriate role models.

This is the sort of "crash program" that the Federal Government should finance, but it may well take a concerted effort by a consortium of foundations to get things started. The SGIM Task Force on Interviewing and Related Skills has made a sound start but sponsorship could be broadened to include the Society of Teachers of Family Medicine, the American Academy of Pediatrics and probably other bodies, including the AAMC. The SGIM deserves great credit for initiating the Task Force but it alone is hard-pressed to do much more with its present resources and there seems little likelihood that general internists alone can develop the critical masses of faculty needed to respond to the apparent void which currently exists. Of all the efforts the medical establishment might make, this one is the most likely to reduce malpractice litigation, improve patient compliance, save money and enhance the medical profession's public image.

BEHAVIORAL SCIENCES

Most of the evidence bearing on the relationship between behavior and health has been assembled in the three volumes referred to previously (Ader and Cohen 1981; Hamburg, Elliott, and Parron 1982; and Ramsey 1988). The second of these, prepared by the Institute of Medicine (IOM) discusses the need to build on the substantial advances, documented in great detail, made by the biobehavioral sciences in recent years. Also set forth are the obstacles to interdisciplinary and interdepartmental (including disciplines and departments outside the medical school) research, as well as the limitations imposed by categorical funding sources and the composition of grant review committees.

Building on the work of the IOM some body should strive to have Congressional hearings held on these matters. The strongest advocates for increases in funds and reallocation of priorities should be the Society of Teachers of Family Medicine, the Society of General Internal Medicine and the American Academy of

Pediatrics. These three bodies would not seek funds for their own training programs, needed as that may be, but rather for support of further fundamental biobehavioral research to broaden the scientific underpinnings for their clinical work and for wider acceptance of the twentieth century model. Success in this endeavor would have the effect of facilitating research by the basic behavioral and biological sciences in support of the efforts of their clinical colleagues in an arena that holds exciting promise for all participants. Those requesting the hearings will need to collaborate carefully, do their homework effectively and lobby constructively. Some foundation should help them in achieving the goal of obtaining large increases in Federal funds for biobehavioral research, especially that which involves integrated laboratory, field and population-based research.

As a consequence of this research, medical students should have increased exposure to the behavioral sciences. If research in the biobehavioral sciences is increased, it is more then likely that behavioral scientists will be asked to teach more, especially in the preclinical years. If steps are taken to insist that the standards for interviewing and communication skills are raised substantially, behavioral scientists will be asked to help even more in the clinical years.

Two other areas require special attention: the sociology and anthropology *of* medicine and the health professions and sociology and anthropology *in* medicine. The first deals with the traditions, culture and practices of the medical and related professions, their institutions and services, and their relationships with patients and populations from their origins to the present, including comparisons with experiences in the cultures of other countries. The second deals with the impact of constructive and deleterious societal and cultural changes on health and disease, with the impact of socioeconomic factors on health and also with the ways in which, for example, traditions and cultural practices mold the ways in which patients express and tolerate pain and disability, label or present their health problems, and respond to interventions from different sources. Although covered sporadically by sociologists and anthropologists working in medical schools, systematic immersion in these bodies of knowledge is not part of every medical student's education; it should be.

In spite of the obvious needs and opportunities, behavioral science departments and units in medical schools continue to have their teaching opportunities limited and their relevance questioned (Institute of Medicine 1983). Once competence in many of the skills taught by behavioral scientists is accepted as a fundamental component of a contemporary medical education it should not take long to set standards. The National Board of Medical Examiners already asks some questions and the Liaison Committee on Medical Education pays some deference to the field in its reviews. The NBME could ask more questions on the final as well as on the Part I examinations and the Liaison Committees could pursue more rigorous questioning during their visits; they should have a behavioral scientist on each review team. If both the NBME and the Liaison Committee act in the public interest to deal with these obvious lacunae in medical education, the medical schools will find a way to sort out their educational priorities. If action is to follow, some body must decide that these matters are important and act accordingly.

PRIMARY CARE

The time is now ripe for an independent body, similar to the Citizens Commission on Graduate Medical Education (1966)—the Millis Commission—to examine the place of primary medical care in the overall health services arrangements in the United States. The central issue to be resolved is whether primary care is just an "add-on" to the real business of medicine designed, for example, to keep state legislators and consumer groups quiet or whether American medical schools should assume collective responsibility for educating and training a primary care sector capable of looking after 90 percent of the population's health problems. In other words, should the bulk of these problems be taken directly to subspecialists of various types or should they be cared for by an appropriately trained generalist? Until this issue is settled and clearly enunciated, there is little prospect that much of the present turmoil can subside.

Unlike the Millis Commission, which used a top-down approach for its deliberations, primarily examining the problems from the teachers' and the profession's perspectives, the new commission should use a bottom-up or population-based approach. For this purpose the members now would have available data from, for example, the National Household Interview Survey, the National Ambulatory Medical Care Survey, the National Hospital Discharge Survey, the Ambulatory Sentinel Practice Network and from large health maintenance organizations, as well as data from national and regional health statistical sources in Britain, Canada, the Netherlands and Finland. Testimony based on twenty years of analysis, demonstration and experience both in the United States and abroad should help to further inform the group. These sources of information and understanding were not available to the Millis Commission.

Some of the basic questions that should be addressed to clarify and amplify the central issue include:

(i) What is the content of primary care practice as defined by the patients who seek it? What are the medical problems brought to this source of care and how are they distributed?

(ii) What types of people enjoy this kind of practice and do it well? What personality characteristics and aptitudes do they possess?

(iii) Would the provision of a strong, appropriately trained cadre of dedicated "general physicians" (i.e., primary care internists, family physicians and general pediatricians), constituting a majority of all physicians, reduce costs and improve the care of patients?

(iv) Would the creation of a new category of "general physician" or "personal physician" be in the public interest? Should encouragement and support be given to the dialogue now under way between groups of general internists and family physicians who are discussing various forms of cooperation and amalgamation? If these moves are deemed desirable, how could they best be brought about?

(v) What are the appropriate balances between generalists and specialists to be sought? If the present arrangements are out of balance, how would we know when they were in balance?

(vi) What undergraduate and postgraduate training is required to obtain and sustain enduring proficiency in the wide range of knowledge and skills needed by the primary care physician?

(vii) How can research in this poorly understood field of primary care best be stimulated? Without a vigorous tradition of productive and credible research can this field survive and does it deserve to survive?

(viii) What changes should be made in the allocation of resources to achieve the goals proposed by the new commission?

If there is a decision to recommend substantial increases in numbers, quality and duration of training as well as changes in the sites for training "general physicians," then extensive attention should be paid to methods for financing these changes; they are likely to be more costly than traditional models, at least in the short term. A voucher system for financing residency training was proposed by The Task Force on Academic Health Centers (1985) but there are other possibilities. The Wickenburg Conference prompted Christian Ramsey to suggest that an "investment model" be developed to finance the cost of postgraduate training in primary care. In such a model the output of the program would be measured by diagnostic tests performed, referrals made and patient days in hospital—more accurate measures of the trainees' accomplishments than mere body counts of trainees produced. After all, the central questions are: How do the graduates perform clinically? What else do they accomplish? Their collective efforts in each training program should be reflected in the savings that accrue to the hospital and its associated health care system; the hypotheses are that in due course the increased costs of training will be offset by the savings in patient care and that in the long run overall savings to the system could be substantial.

If all these suggestions have merit then one or more foundations will probably have to take the first steps to appoint, staff and charge an appropriate panel—a panel composed primarily of lay persons above the fray. As in the case of the Millis Commission, use of the British Royal Commission format should contribute materially to the credibility of its recommendations.

PLACEBO AND HAWTHORNE EFFECTS

The relative importance of the placebo and Hawthorne effects, and of Factor X, seems unsettled in many minds. Are they as ubiquitous as some claim? Do they constitute a potentially significant therapeutic modality? If these factors are as important as much available evidence suggests then they may exert their influence throughout the health care enterprise, not only during primary care encounters but also during tertiary care diagnostic endeavors, during therapeutic maneuvers of all types, and in the course of providing family, community and social support as well as many public health services. Enthusiasm, earnest intentions, desire to do "good," "black boxes" of diverse types and organized efforts to "help" and "care" should be properly identified, called by their correct names, and paid for appropriately.

The placebo, Hawthorne and X factors should be distinguished from the intrinsic "objective" qualities of the maneuver they accompany; they may be just as important therapeutically as the latter. But how important are these effects? If indeed, there are associations or more specific relationships suggested from population-based, clinical or laboratory investigations, what is known about how these influences are mediated through neuroendocrine, neuropeptide, immunological and other systems? If there is some credible evidence available, what additional research is needed to settle any outstanding issues?

Central to this exercise is the notion of the physician herself or himself as a primary therapeutic agent—as well as a listener, counselor and teacher. A clear understanding of the role and importance of these factors should do much to clarify the need for any changes that may be deemed appropriate in the allocation of resources for research, education and services.

Some organization should conduct an inquiry into the role of the placebo, Hawthorne and Factor X effects; the likelihood is slight that the evidence could be adequately sifted and evaluated in the course of a short conference or symposium—a more extensive examination is justified by the currently available evidence. The Institute of Medicine would be an appropriate body. During the recent extensive examination of the biobehavioral sciences, little or no attention appears to have been paid to this important sphere of clinical practice (Hamburg, Elliott, and Parron 1982). It should not be difficult to assemble a panel to prepare a report similar to others developed in related fields.

THE LITERATE PHYSICIAN

The allegedly narrow education of many physicians is said to be reflected in the limited understanding they seem to have of the power of literature, history, the arts and scholarship generally to enhance our understanding of human affairs and the human condition. When suggestions are made, such as C. P. Snow's (1973), that "there ought to be a literary component throughout the course of medical education," the cry goes out, "don't add more courses to the curriculum!" First, we should determine the facts. Are physicians as a group, compared to say, lawyers, engineers, accountants and business executives more stunted in their exposure to the humanities? Dr. Odegaard's examination of the record suggests that many leaders of the medical establishment appear to have a limited understanding of how our present turmoil relates to what has gone before. To know more about the dimensions of the problem should be helpful; current popular books suggest that cultural illiteracy is endemic in America. If necessary, the facts could be established with a competently conducted survey. Here is another opportunity for the AAMC.

Supposing physicians as a group are as unenlightened as the rest of the citizenry, should we not want this country's medical profession to have a deeper appreciation of the enduring dilemmas, ambiguities and uncertainties that our forebears experienced, and that continue to surround us, in our efforts to improve our common lot? There are approaches that could be adopted other than simply "more courses."

1. The AAMC could recommend or even urge that undergraduate proficiency in the humanities (as well as in the behav-

ioral sciences) be accorded equal weight with proficiency in the natural sciences for admission to medical school. For those who believe the MCAT is an instrument useful in the selection process, a module could be constructed to assess knowledge and appreciation in this domain.

After all, available evidence suggests that even students who *major* in the humanities or the social sciences do just as well in medical school as those who major in the natural sciences. The evidence is ambiguous but there appears to be no evidence that those students with high grade point averages (GPAs) in natural science subjects do any better than those with high GPAs in nonscience subjects (Woodward and McAuley 1983). But, of course, that is not really the issue. The central question is how do they perform as physicians?

2. The AAMC could commission a suitable group to prepare bibliographies, including shorter and longer versions, on such topics as: the history of ideas in science, medicine and health services; evolution of the scientific method; biographies of physicians; health and disease in fiction, art, drama and poetry; physicians as artists and authors. A publisher might be encouraged to bring out inexpensive paperback editions of these "classics," possibly sold through monthly book club subscriptions. Medical school libraries could be encouraged to place the collections in readily accessible locations.

LABELING

The labeling of health problems, nosology as the generic topic, and nomenclature and classification as the applied topics, have been discussed above. On the one hand, we have the dehumanizing, denigrating and pejorative labels increasingly used by house staff and students and, on the other, we have had, until recently, an inadequate nomenclature and classification for use in primary care. Some would say the ICD is also inadequate for much secondary level community hospital care, and there is growing dissatisfaction with the DRG system among physicians, hospital administrators, politicians and the public. In particular there are no traditions of providing social and psychological labels or "diagnoses," in addition to the biological; nor are there traditions for stating the physician's assessment of the severity of the patient's illness and the patient's functional status at various points in the course of management.

Much work has been done in these areas, particularly in the development of the *International Classification of Primary Care* (Lamberts and Wood 1987). Acceptance of the twentieth century model is likely to be facilitated if we provide a reasonably rich but appropriate language with which all of the patient's problems and medical interventions during the course of an episode of illness can be properly identified, recorded, and counted. Once the distributions of the components of care are known, and the evidence supports the need, the case can be made effectively to change reimbursement schemes and resource allocation priorities.

Information is power and there is every reason to believe that changes in nomenclature and classifications will be fiercely resisted in some circles. The time is now ripe for a foundation or a consortium of interested professionals to convene a body to examine the generic public policy, educational and practice issues that surround our current labeling systems and the innovative ideas embodied in the *International Classification of Primary Care*. If classification is an essential tool for any scientific endeavor then the underlying assumptions and characteristics of the classifications employed must make a difference.

Health Information and Analysis Units

The Institute of Medicine's report on *Medical Education and Societal Needs: A Planning Report for the Health Professions* (1983), recommended establishing a national Agenda Group on Education of Health Professionals. This is a powerful idea but for a presumably science-based enterprise there was remarkably little said about the need to use population-based information or even data of any kind for guiding decisions of the Agenda Group. As yet another top-down operation, "the group would be a continuing monitor of events, trends, quality, critical thinking, and conceptualization about health professional education both at the national and state level." "Extensive consultation and collaboration with leaders of national, regional, and state professional organizations and educational institutions, and with policymakers" was advocated. Elsewhere in the Report there was a recommendation that the group "identify topics in need of further data gathering and/or analysis," but the notion that determination of people's individual and aggregate problems and needs might be the basis for setting priorities and developing education, research and service policies appears to have escaped the Panel. There is much more that can be done.

A similar innovation not at the national or state (or provincial) levels but at the institutional level is to be found at McMaster University in Canada. Funded by the Ontario Ministry of Health, a Health Information and Analysis Unit has been established within its Health Sciences Center (Neufeld 1987). This unit is fashioned after a suggestion made at the Montebello Conference on *Health in the '8os and '9os and its Impact on Health Sciences Education* (1983). The suggestion made at that meeting was that every vice-chancellor of health sciences (or whatever the local title is) should have an "intelligence" unit attached to her or his office. The unit's task would be to keep the vice-chancellor, the faculty, students and the public informed about the health status of the population served, changes in its status, especially compared to other geographic jurisdictions; to monitor major advances in medicine, medical education and health services, new interventions and technology; and to assess their potential impact on the health sciences centers, other related institutions, the health professions and society. Newsletters and material suitable for the media would be distributed in timely fashion. Acting as a combination ombudsman and beacon light, this Unit would not undertake most of these data acquisition activities itself but would gather information from diverse sources and, where appropriate, encourage others to collect or seek the necessary information. The unit would conduct secondary analyses and interpretations to guide the faculty's overall institutional research, educational and service priorities. In the case of research, there should be no inherent conflict between institutional responses to societal needs and individual investigator's responses to curiosity.

More broadly this unit should help the area's health institutions and professions to define their tasks with increasing specificity. In so doing they could make explicit to the community what medicine can provide, what other agencies can reasonably be expected to do, what the citizenry have to do for themselves and where more research is needed. Such matters as patient-physician relations and communication, knowledge of the placebo, Hawthorne and X effects, costs and benefits of new capital intensive technology and of high volume, low-cost interventions of limited benefit, and knowledge and attitudes about preventive practices would be among the many factors mentioned, in addition to seeing that statistical information about the distribution of health problems and associated disability, and what was done about them, is available on a timely basis. The technology for doing all this is now available and McMaster proposes to apply it. Other medical schools and health sciences centers may wish to introduce similar innovations. State health departments would be a reasonable source of funding but foundations might help with the initial start-up costs.

THE THREE SCANDALS

Finally we should deal with what I have identified as the three scandals discussed at Wickenburg. In order to do that effectively we need first to be assured about the actual prevalence of each of these alleged practices and second to develop a consensus that they are unacceptable.

1. The use of demeaning, dehumanizing, denigrating and pejorative language by resident physicians and students to describe patients and their problems should be stopped. First amendment rights of these two groups would not be abridged by deans, department heads and hospital administrators embarking on a national campaign to stop such practices. Open discussions of the matter at annual meetings of the AAMC and the American Hospital Association should start the process. Although negative sanctions could be taken, positive incentives might prove more

effective—especially if accompanied by widespread publicity. A series of ten or more well-advertised, substantial annual awards (i.e., $25,000 or more for each hospital) might be given for all the chief residents of the major clinical services to share. The winners would be required to provide a panel of lay judges with evidence that their institution has "cleaned up its act!" The best documented submissions would receive the awards; ingenuity would be encouraged.

2. Next there is the alleged failure of attending physicians to visit the bedsides of the patients on their teaching services, talk to them and undertake appropriate examinations in the course of "rounds." The Association of American Medical Colleges (AAMC), together with its Council of Teaching Hospitals, should mount a properly designed national survey to determine the actual state of affairs, bearing in mind that the Wickenburg Conference was told that such bedside visits were made to only 20 to 30 percent of patients (presumably "new" patients) on the teaching services. The results should be debated in a forum that includes representatives from medical faculties, physicians in practice, medical students, residents and representatives of the public. Once the importance of the findings for patient care and medical education have been determined they should be widely disseminated. If changes are in order, the AAMC, the Liaison Committee on Medical Education and the residency review committees should take remedial action to change standards and performance.

3. The third matter concerns the need to assess "integrity," "respect," and "compassion." These aspects of physicians' fitness to practice medicine should be assessed in medical school. If the AAMC cannot motivate the medical schools to undertake this task themselves then the National Board of Medical Examiners should set the standards and evaluate the students at the time of graduation. The complexities of the task were reviewed in the IOM Report on *Medical Education and Societal Needs: A Planning Report for the Health Professions* (1983) but the matter seems too serious to neglect any longer. Once the public gets wind of the notion that these qualities are still in question and

that they are only assessed when the physician is about to take final specialty board examinations—after perhaps ten or eleven years of formal education, much at public expense—there is bound to be a substantial clamor for prompt reform. A conspiracy of silence is unlikely to be a satisfactory response.

CONCLUSION

THE DISCUSSION AT WICKENBURG focused on the importance of broadening both the information base for understanding our patients' problems and the framework for interpreting what we learn. The argument for broadening our perspectives is derived both from historical appreciation of the wide spectrum of scholarly and scientific approaches to eliciting and interpreting information bearing on these matters, and from the content of that information.

At no point during the Conference were the extraordinary advances in understanding the biological aspects of health and disease questioned, nor were there any doubts expressed about medicine's remarkable technological advances—advances from which a number of participants had benefited personally. These matters are not at issue; we need more, not less, first-rate biomedical research.

The issues raised in *Dear Doctor* and discussed at Wickenburg have been of interest, as I have tried to show, for almost half a century, to many physicians, fundamental and applied medical scientists, behavioral scientists, other scholars and the public. Contrary to the impression some of those now in office and in other positions of leadership may have, these issues are not new. They concern the optimal means by which advances in biomedicine and medical technology can be extended and expanded beyond anything yet imagined. Are there ways in which we could broaden the application of contemporary biomedicine, stimulate further research using a more inclusive model and develop new interventions—not only within biological systems but also within behavioral, social, institutional and even political systems? What can possibly be lost by embracing biobehavioral research more aggressively, by listening to our patients more carefully, by increasing our sensitivity to the influences of psychological and social factors on health and disease and by organizing our educational efforts and our health services so that they respond to an array of needs wider than the biological?

In all of this we need to develop a national dialogue that helps our profession to define its task primarily from our patients' and the public's perspectives—not primarily from our own perspectives. The notion that "doctors know best" is no longer acceptable—anywhere! What can possibly be lost by adopting patient-oriented and population-based perspectives in defining our collective task? The prospect of accomplishing this can be enhanced only by the broadest possible appreciation of the human condition—an appreciation that requires understanding and wisdom derived from the humanities, and knowledge and skills derived as much from the behavioral as from the natural sciences.

We should start the dialogue by discussing changes in the requirements for medical school admission. Why should we not accord as much weight to competence in the humanities and the behavioral sciences as to the natural sciences? Medical school faculties should recognize that physicians, more than most, require: opportunities for full development of both left and right brain functions, the qualities of integrity, respect and compassion, and a broad understanding of the evolution of their profession within the context of man's search for a healthier and happier society. Why should not the behavioral and population-based sciences be accorded equal emphasis with the biological sciences in the preclinical years? Should not the scientific method as a way of thinking about our patients' problems and the population's problems permeate the entire curriculum? The hallmarks of sound study designs, the benefits of measurement, and the importance of critical appraisal of the medical literature, all deserve continual emphasis, but so also do the rules of evidence and the laws of logic as they apply to historical and clinical information elicited from the patient and the family. Progress has been slow or imperceptible on most of these fronts. Failure to obtain evidence or to examine its credibility is just as serious an infringement of the canons of science and scholarship as selection of the types of evidence to be considered. More—not less—science, and more—not less—"scientific effort" (Flexner's phrase) are needed.

The hope is that the dialogue started at Wickenburg will expand and improve the quality of muted discussions during the past fifty years. The present turmoil engulfing medicine and the sea change that swirls about us require that we engage in this dialogue on a national scale. What exactly is the "business of medicine" as Charles Odegaard phrases it, or the "task of medicine" as I term it? Much has been accomplished but there is much more to do; our task is to start the process of change. Success is most likely to ensue if we listen to our patients and their families. Listening to our patients may not always be sufficient but it is always necessary. If there is doubt, why not resort to the evidence?

REFERENCES

References marked with an asterisk may be of special interest to those who wish to explore these matters further.

*Abercrombie, M.L.J. *The Anatomy of Judgment*. New York, Basic Books Inc., 1960.

Ader, R. and Cohen, N. eds. *Psychoneuroimmunology*. New York, Academic Press, 1981.

Aldrich, C.K. and Mendkoff, E. Relocation of the Aged and Disabled: A Mortality Study. *J Amer Geriatrics Soc* 11:185–194, 1963.

American Board of Internal Medicine. *A Guide to Awareness and Evaluation of Humanistic Qualities in the Internist*. Portland, Ore., American Board of Internal Medicine, 1985.

Angell, M. Disease as a Reflection of the Psyche. Editorial. *New Eng J Med* 312:1570–1572, 1985.

Bailer, J.C. III and Mosteller, F., eds. *Medical Uses of Statistics*. Waltham, Mass., NEJM Books, 1986.

Balint, M. The Doctor, His Patient and the Illness. *Lancet* 1:683–688, 1955.

*Balint, M. *The Doctor, His Patient and the Illness*. London, Pitman Medical Publishing Company, Ltd., 1957.

Beale, N. and Nethercott, S. Job-loss and Family Morbidity: A Study of Factory Closure. *J Royal Coll Gen Pract* 35:510–514, 1985.

Bertalanffy, L. von. Problems of General System Theory. *Human Biology* 23:302–312, 1951.

Bingham, W. V. D. and Moore, B. V. *How to Interview*. New York, Harper and Row, 1924.

Bird, B. *Talking with Patients*. Philadelphia, J. B. Lipincott Company, 1955.

Bisht, D. B. *The Spiritual Dimension of Health*. New Delhi, Directorate General of Health Services, Government of India, 1985.

Blundell, W. E. When the Patient Takes Charge: The Consumer Movement Comes to Medical Care. *Wall Street Journal*, Section 4:1–44, April 24, 1987.

Broadhead, W. E., Kaplan, B. H., James, S. A. et al: The Epidemiologic Evidence for a Relationship Between Social Support and Health. *Amer J Epid* 117:521–537, 1983.

*Brody, H. *Placebos and the Philosophy of Medicine: Clinical, Conceptual and Ethical Issues*. Chicago, The University of Chicago Press, 1980.

Bruer, J. T. and Warren, K. S. Liberal Arts and the Premedical Curriculum. *J A M A* 245:364–366, 1981.

*Cannon, W.B. *The Wisdom of the Body*. New York, W. W. Norton, 1932.

Cassel, J., Patrick, R. and Jenkins, D. J. Epidemiological Analysis of the Health Implications of Culture Change: A Conceptual Model. *Ann New York Acad Sci* 84:938–949, 1960.

Cassell, E. J. *Talking with Patients*, Volume 1, *The Theory of Doctor-Patient Communication*, Volume 2, *Clinical Technique*. Cambridge, Mass., MIT Press, 1985.

Chandra, V., Szklo, M., Goldberg, R. et al. The Impact of Marital Status on Survival After An Acute Myocardial Infarction: A Population-Based Study. *Amer J Epid* 117:320–325, 1983.

Chong, J.P., Neufeld, V., Oates, M.J. et al. The Selection of Priority Problems and Conditions: An Approach to Curriculum Design in Medical Education. 1987 (Submitted for Publication).

Ciocco, A. On the Interdependence of the Length of Life of Husband and Wife. *Human Biology* 13:505–525, 1941.

Citizens Commission on Graduate Medical Education. *The*

Graduate Education of Physicians. Chicago, American Medical Association, 1966.

Cohen-Cole, S. A.: On Teaching the New (and Old) Psychobiology in Friedman, C. P. and Purcell, E. F.: *The New Biology and Medical Education: Merging the Biological, Information and Cognitive Sciences.* New York, Josiah Macy Jr. Foundation, 1983.

College of General Practitioners (Working Party on Records). Continuing Observation and Recording of Morbidity. *J Coll Gen Pract* 1:107, 1958.

Conett, R., Tamarin, F. M., Wogalter, D. et al. Liqueur Lung. *New Eng J Med* 316:348–349, 1987.

*Dawson, W. *Interim Report on the Future Provision of Medical and Allied Services* (Command 693, United Kingdom Ministry of Health, Consultative Council on Medical and Allied Services). London, His Majesty's Stationery Office, 1920 and Reprinted in Saward, E. W., ed. *The Regionalization of Personal Health Services,* New York, Prodist, 1975.

*DeVries, M. J. *The Redemption of the Intangible in Medicine.* London, Institute of Psychosynthesis, 1981.

Donnelly, W. J. Medical Language as Symptom: Doctor Talk in Teaching Hospitals. *Pers Biol and Med* 30:81–94, 1986.

Drossman, D. A. The Physician and the Patient: Review of Psychosocial Gastrointestinal Literature with an Integrated Approach to the Patient, in Sleisenger, M. H. and Fordtran, J. S., eds. *Gastrointestinal Disease: Physiology, Diagnosis, Management,* Fourth Edition. Philadelphia, J. P. Lipincott Company, 1987.

Easterbrook, G. The Revolution in Medicine. *Newsweek,* January 26, 1987:40–74.

Egeland, J. A., Gerhard, D. S., Pauls, D. L. et al. Bipolar Affective Disorders Linked to DNA Markers on Chromosome II. *Nature* 325:783–787, 1987.

Eliot, T. S. *Collected Poems 1909–1962.* The Rock. New York, Harcourt, Brace & World, Inc., 1963.

Engle, A. *Perspectives in Health Planning*. London, The Athlone Press, 1968.

Engel, G. L. Sudden and Rapid Death During Psychological Stress. *Ann Int Med* 74:771–782, 1971.

*Engel, G. L. The Need for a New Medical Model: A Challenge for Biomedicine. *Science* 196:129–136, 1977.

*Faber, K. *Nosography: The Evolution of Clinical Medicine in Modern Times*, Second Edition, Revised. New York, Paul B. Hoeber, Inc., Reprinted by AMES Press, Inc., New York, 1978.

*Feinstein, A. R. The Intellectual Crisis in Clinical Science: Medaled Models and Muddled Metal. *Pers Biol and Med* 30:215–230, 1987.

Finnish Ministry of Social Affairs and Health. *Health Policy Report by the Government of Finland*. Helsinki, May 1985.

Fletcher, R. H., Fletcher, S. W., and Wagner, E. H. *Clinical Epidemiology: The Essentials*. Baltimore, Williams and Wilkins, 1982.

Flexner, A. *Medical Education: A Comparative Study*. New York, The Macmillan Company, 1925.

*Flexner, A. *Universities: American, English, German*. New York, Oxford University Press, 1930.

Forbes, J. F. and McGregor, A. Male Unemployment and Cause-specific Mortality in Postwar Scotland. *Internat J Health Serv* 17:233–240, 1987.

*Foss, L. and Rothenberg, K. *The Second Medical Revolution: From Biomedicine to Infomedicine*. Boston, Shambhala Publications and Random House, 1987.

*Fox, T. F. The Personal Doctor and His Relation to the Hospital. *Lancet* 1:743–760, 1960.

GPEP Report: *Physicians for the Twenty-first Century*. The Panel on the General Professional Education of the Physician and College Preparation for Medicine. Washington, D.C., Association of American Medical Colleges, 1984.

Green, L. A., Wood, M., Becker, L. et al. The Ambulatory Sentinel Practice Network: Purpose, Methods and Policies. *J Fam Med* 18:275–280, 1984.

Haggerty, R. J. Stress and Illness in Children. *Bull N Y Acad Med* 62:707–718, 1987.

Hamburg, D. A., Elliott, G. R. and Parron, D. L. eds. *Health and Behavior: Frontiers of Research in the Biobehavioral Sciences*, Report of a Study by the Institute of Medicine. Washington, D.C., National Academy Press, 1982.

Helsing, K. J., Comstock, G. W. and Szklo, M. Causes of Death in a Widowed Population. *Amer J Epid* 116:524–532, 1982.

Hilfiker, D. *Healing the Wounds: A Physician Looks at His Work.* New York, Penguin Books, 1987.

Hoaglin, D. C., Light, R. J., McPeek, B. et al. *Data for Decisions.* Cambridge, Massachusetts, Abt Books, 1982.

Institute of Medicine: *Medical Education and Societal Needs: A Planning Report for the Health Professions.* Washington, D.C., National Academy Press, 1983.

Inui, T. S., Yourtree, E. L. and Williamson, J. W. Improved Outcome in Hypertension After Physician Tutorials. *Ann Int Med* 84:646–651, 1976.

Jaco, G. E. ed. *Patients, Physicians and Illness: Sourcebook in Behavioral Science and Medicine.* Glencoe, Illinois, The Free Press, 1958.

Kahn, R. L., and Cannell, C. F. *The Dynamics of Interviewing: Theory, Technique and Cases.* New York, John Wiley & Sons, Inc., 1957.

Kark, S. L. *The Practice of Community-Oriented Primary Health Care.* New York, Appleton-Century Crofts, 1981.

Katz, J. *The Silent World of Doctor and Patient.* New York, The Free Press, 1984.

Kuhn, T. S. *The Structure of Scientific Revolutions*, Second Edition. Chicago, University of Chicago Press, 1970.

*Lamberts, H. and Wood, M., eds. *International Classification of Primary Care*, Oxford, Oxford University Press, 1987.

Last, J. M. The Iceberg. *Lancet* 2:28–31, 1963.

Lee, P. V. *Medical Schools and the Changing Times: Nine Case Reports on Experimentation in Medical Education, 1950–1960*. Evanston, Illinois, Association of American Medical Colleges, 1962.

Lipkin, M. *The Care of Patients*, Revised Edition. New Haven, Yale University Press, 1987.

Lipkin, M., Jr. and Kupka, K. *Psychosocial Factors Affecting Health*. New York, Praeger Scientific, 1982.

Lipkin, M., Jr., Quill, T. E., and Napodano, R. J. The Medical Interview: A Core Curriculum for Residencies in Internal Medicine. *Ann Int Med* 100:277–284, 1984.

*Mackenzie, J. *The Future of Medicine*. London, Henry Frowde and Hodder & Stoughton, 1919.

*Mair, A. *Sir James Mackenzie, M.D., 1853–1925, General Practitioner*. Edinburgh and London, Churchill Livingstone, pp 274–275, 1973.

Manton, K. G. and Vertrees, J. C. The Use of Grade of Membership Analysis to Evaluate and Modify Diagnosis-related Groups. *Medical Care* 22:1067–1082, 1984.

Mayo, E. *The Human Problems of an Industrial Civilization*. New York, The Macmillan Company, 1933.

Moser, K. A., Fox, A. J. and Jones, D. R. Unemployment and Mortality in the OPCS Longitudinal Study. *Lancet* 2:1324–1329, 1984.

Needham, J. New Advances in Chemistry and Biology of Organized Growth. *Proc Roy Soc Med* 29, Part II:31, 1936.

Neufeld, V. R. Priority Health Problems in Medical Education: Progress Report of Task Force II, McMaster University, Ham-

ilton, Canada (Mimeographed). Faculty of Medicine, Rijksuniversiteit Limburg, Maastricht, The Netherlands, Network of
Community-Oriented Educational Institutions for Health Sciences, 1987.

Neufeld, V. R. Personal Communication, 1987.

Novack, D. H. Therapeutic Aspects of the Clinical Encounter. *J
Gen Int Med* 1987 (In press).

Nutting, P. A., ed. *Community-Oriented Primary Care: From Prin-
ciple to Practice* (HRSA Publication No. HRS-A-PE 86-1).
Washington, D.C., U.S. Department of Health and Human
Services, 1987.

★Odegaard, C. E. *Dear Doctor—A Personal Letter to a Physician*.
Menlo Park, The Henry J. Kaiser Family Foundation, 1986.

Office of Technology Assessment. *Diagnosis Related Groups
(DRGs) and the Medicare Program: Implications for Medical Technol-
ogy*. Washington, D.C., Congress of the United States, Office of
Technology Assessment, 1983.

★Pan American Health Organization. Prospective Analysis of
Medical Education: A Self-Evaluatory Methodology. Human
Resources Series No. 72 (Mimeographed). Washington, D.C.,
Pan American Health Organization, 1987.

Payer, L. *Beyond the Second Opinion: A Quizzical Inquiry Concerning French, German, English and U.S. Medicine*. New York,
Henry Holt, 1988 (In press).

Pearse, I. H. *The Quality of Life: The Peckham Approach to Human
Ethology*. Edinburgh, Scottish Academic Press, 1979.

Pearse, I. H. and Crocker, L. H. *The Peckham Experiment: A
Study in The Living Structure of Society*. London, George Allen &
Unwin, Ltd., 1943.

Popper, K. R. *The Logic of Scientific Discovery*. New York, Science Editions, Inc., 1961.

Querido, A. Forecast and Follow-up: An Investigation into the

Clinical, Social and Mental Factors Determining the Results of Hospital Treatment. *Brit J Prev Social Med* 13:33–49, 1959.

Querido, A. *The Efficiency of Medical Care*. Leiden, H. E. Stenfert Kroese N.V., 1963.

Ramsey, C. N., Jr. ed. *Family Systems in Medicine*. New York, Guilford Press, 1988 (In press).

Richter, C. P. On the Phenomenon of Sudden Death in Animals and Man. *Psychosom Med* 19:191–198, 1957.

Rogers, C. R. *Counselling and Psychotherapy*. Boston, Houghton Mifflin Co., 1942.

Romanucci-Ross, L., Moerman, D. E. and Trancredi, L. R., eds. *The Anthropology of Medicine: From Culture to Method*. South Hadley, Mass., Bergin & Garvey Publishers Inc., 1983.

Rosser, W. W. and Beaulieu, M. Institutional Objectives for Medical Education that Relates to the Community. *Can Med Assoc J* 130:683–689, 1984.

Sackett, D. L., Haynes, R. B. and Tugwell, P. *Clinical Epidemiology: A Basic Science for Clinical Medicine*. Boston, Little Brown and Company, 1985.

Seldin, D. W. Presidential Address: The Boundaries of Medicine. *Trans Assoc Am Phys* 94:75–84, 1981.

Sheldrake, R. *A New Science of Life: The Hypothesis of Formative Causation*. London, Blond & Biggs Ltd., 1981.

*Shorter, E. *Bedside Manners: The Troubled History of Doctors and Patients*. New York, Simon and Schuster, 1985.

Siegel, B. S. *Love, Medicine & Miracles: Lessons Learned About Self-Healing from a Surgeon's Experience With Exceptional Patients*. New York, Harper and Row, 1987.

Smith, R. C. Unrecognized Responses and Feelings of Residents and Fellows During Interviews with Patients. *J Med Educ* 61:982–984, 1986.

Smuts, J. C. *Holism and Evolution.* London, The Macmillan Company, 1926.

Snow, C. P. *The Two Cultures and the Scientific Revolution.* Cambridge, Cambridge University Press, 1959.

Snow, C. P. Human Care. *J A M A* 225:617–621, 1973.

*Squires, B. P., ed. *Proceedings of the Conference on Health in the '80s and '90s and Its Impact on Health Sciences.* Toronto, Council of Ontario Universities, 1983.

Stevenson, I: Scientists with Half-closed Minds. *Harper's Magazine,* November 1958, pp 66–71.

Stevenson, I. The End of Patient Abuse in Medical Care. *Virginia Quart Rev* 61:565–583, 1985.

Stillman, P., Brown, D., Redfield, D. et al. Construct Validation of the Arizona Clinical Interview Rating Scale. *Educ Psycho Meas* 77:1031–1038, 1977.

Stillman, P. L., Swanson, D. B., Smee, S. et al. Assessing Clinical Skills of Residents with Standardized Patients. *Ann Int Med* 105:762–771, 1986.

Szasz, T. S. and Hollender, M. C. A Contribution to the Philosophy of Medicine. *Arch Int Med* 97:585–592, 1956.

Task Force on Academic Health Centers. *Prescription for Change.* New York, N. Y., The Commonwealth Fund, 1985.

The Economist. Schools Brief—The Philosophy of Science. 303:(April 25)70–71, 1987.

White, K. L. Primary Care Research and the New Epidemiology. *J Fam Med* 1976;3:5–580, 1976.

White, K. L. Restructuring the International Classification of Diseases: Need for a New Paradigm. *J Fam Med* 21:17–20, 1985.

White, K. L., Williams, T. F. and Greenberg, B. G. The Ecology of Medical Care. *New Eng J Med* 265:885–892, 1961.

Wolf, S. *Talking with the Patient*. New York, Paul B. Hoeber, Medical Book Division of Harper Brothers, 1952.

Wood, M. What is NAPCRG? *J Fam Med* 12;23–24, 1981.

Woodward, C.A., and McAuley, R.G. Can the Academic Background of Medical Graduates be Detected During Internship? *Can Med Assoc J* 129:567–569, 1983.

Woodward, C. A. Assessing the Relationship Between Medical Education and Subsequent Performance. *Assess Eval High Educ* 9:19–29, 1984.

World Health Organization: *Manual of the International Statistical Classification of Diseases*, Injuries and Causes of Death (ICD), Ninth Revision. Geneva, World Health Organization, 1977.

Ziman, J. *Reliable Knowledge: An Exploration of the Grounds for Belief in Science*. Cambridge, Cambridge University Press, 1978.

APPENDICES

TOWARDS AN IMPROVED DIALOGUE

by

Charles E. Odegaard

My purpose in this essay is to provide some introductory remarks about a new dialogue in which hopefully we shall be collectively engaged. I hope that we may think of this dialogue as
initiating a national seminar. By choosing the word seminar I
mean to connote a joint learning process in which each participant, perhaps in varying degrees, is both a learner and a teacher,
a listener and also a contributor to the ensuing discussion.

I see no indication of disrespect for faculty if concerned professors, chairmen, deans, or presidents arrange from time to
time for faculty to go back to school, perhaps not for lectures,
but for a joint critical review of our established ways in a seminar
in which all participants can be learners as well as teachers. Indeed, the very deep-seated drive within the modern university
toward specialization and subspecialization in the face of an obviously complex universe around us—and within us—makes
desirable such opportunities for determining course corrections
in our pursuit of science and learning and our subsequent design
of instructional programs. Indeed, the litany about challenging
new problems confronting the profession of medicine which I
heard in the plenary sessions of the last annual meeting of the
AAMC in New Orleans, suggests that this is hardly the time
simply for reaffirmation of the status quo in medical education.
Rather, it would seem to be a time for the faculties of medical
schools themselves to go back to school for a reconsideration of
their presuppositions and curricular efforts.

I regret to say that such a review at this time still seems to me
to be timely despite the fact that the most elaborate and official
review of medical education in several decades was completed as
recently as 1984. I refer of course to the Report of the Panel on
the General Professional Education of the Physician and College
Preparation for Medicine appointed by the Association of

American Medical Colleges, the report entitled *Physicians for the Twenty-First Century.*[1] This report devoted considerable attention to the methods of teaching in medical schools, both criticizing pedagogical methods currently in use and recommending substantial changes in *how* to teach medicine. Its criticisms and recommendations surely deserve serious consideration by medical school faculties. As to the matter of content in the teaching of future physicians, Dr. John A. D. Cooper, President of the AAMC, stated in his afterword to the Panel's Report:

> Any comprehensive examination of medical education is destined to be compared with the 1910 Flexner report to the Carnegie Foundation for the Advancement of Teaching. That report established a specific benchmark against which all programs of medical education could be measured, by advocating that a firm scientific base be combined with practical clinical experience within a university setting. Thus, the Flexnerian form of medical education was established, and this form of medical education has remained essentially unchanged for 70 years.

One cannot escape the conclusion that in this Report the Flexnerian form of medical education with its exclusive concentration on disease as simply a malfunction of the organs and tissues of the body interpreted in the light of findings based on the biological, chemical, and physical sciences was accepted without the need for any comment. The Panel in its Report simply did not subject it to critical review.

Perhaps one should not be surprised that the Panel did not really raise as an issue for review the content of medical education. Its behavior is just another indication of the degree to which the Flexnerian doctrine still survives as an establishment doctrine, the orthodox view as to the intellectual content of medicine held by a great majority of medical educators and possibly the medical profession.

That the profession of medicine has gained enormously in the efficacy of its care of patients by acquiring a cognitive base in bioscience is not to be questioned. The utility of bioscience to medicine is not raised as an issue here. But there is a question which has been raised increasingly in the last three decades as to whether bioscience is a sufficient base for medical education. This rising, if still relatively weak heresy, expands the knowledge base of medicine to include, in the terminology suggested by Dr. George Engel, the biopsychosocial sciences, which has now gained some currency, at least among the heretics. Let me call your particular attention to the fact that the protagonists for psychosocial aspects found in medical practice do not regard them merely as add-ons, supplemental elements, in addition to biological aspects, but as interactive aspects.

There is then no hidden agenda here. We hope to stimulate opportunities for discussion of the biopsychosocial concept of illness and disease as an improved cognitive base for better, more effective medical diagnosis and therapy for treatment of patients, for an improved clinical practice of medicine. Let me repeat the reference to clinical practice. Medicine is a practical profession. The object of physicians is to help sick persons, patients. For this the physician has need of knowledge found to be relevant to clinical practice. At least three generations ago some physicians themselves began to go to German universities to study under bioscientific professors to acquire knowledge which they could then apply to the practice of medicine. In time there was less need for physicians themselves to go abroad as they gained access within medical schools in the United States to bioscientists either imported from abroad or by 1900 trained within American universities, so-called basic scientists who could provide physicians with access to scientific knowledge which they could then apply to clinical cases. Over close to a century physicians in this country have had an opportunity to become closely associated within medical schools with basic scientists, possessed of knowledge in the biological sciences. Physicians themselves have had opportunities over decades in which to build up research competence in applying relevant bioscience to clinical problems in medical practice. They have in fact learned about, and learned to make applications to medicine of, a relatively restricted area of knowledge pursued in the modern university.

Here is where we English-speakers run into a peculiar problem of language. Science is a troublesome word. It is derived from the Latin *scientia*, which generally means knowledge—in modern times, knowledge gained by human reasoning, based upon induction, our careful analysis of givens resulting from our sensory and bodily contacts with the here and now world around us. *Science* in French, and *Wissenschaft*, its equivalent in German, are applied to knowledge so gained about nature and also about man as an individual and as a social creature. Hence, one can speak in French about *les sciences humaines*. *Wissenschaft* in German usage applies equally to similar rational studies of man as well as nature. For reasons of history which I have tried to explain in *Dear Doctor*,[2] science in English has been largely restricted to knowledge about nature, the natural world.

Since physicians in general have had far more exposure to experiences in the biosciences than in the humanities and social sciences, and since you are physicians, please permit me to make a few remarks about the latter groups of disciplines which I hope may be helpful to our discussions here.

You will recall that the National Academy of Sciences was established by federal charter in 1863 during the Civil War to facilitate the provision to the U.S. government of advice from natural scientists about military technology and the care of the wounded associated with the conduct of war. As the prospect of U.S. involvement in World War I emerged, the National Research Council was established in 1916 as an arm of the Academy to improve the availability to the government of such scientific advice. With the defeat of the enemy at the end of World War I the heads of the four successful powers faced a different set of problems, the need to make decisions about territorial divisions and assignments in Asia and Africa as well as Europe. To make such decisions, they needed advice from scholars familiar with the history, languages, cultures, and politics of many peoples on planet Earth. A considerable number of such scholars from different countries were brought together in Versailles as advisors to the treaty makers. These scholars from various lands, when not engaged in advising the heads of the victorious states, fell to discussing the need for international scholarly projects relevant to the study of man and his history which could be established under an organized international body. They therefore established the International Union of Academies headquartered in Brussels, with which national bodies could become affiliates. While many other countries had appropriately organized national academies, no such organization existed in the United States. The membership of the National Academy of Sciences was obviously not relevant for such a purpose. In the United States, however, there were a number of national societies devoted to studies of one or another aspect of man and his culture. The returning American scholars therefore proceeded to organize in 1919 the American Council of Learned Societies—to give it the full title—Devoted to Humanistic Studies (ACLS). Since in English usage "scientific" societies were concerned with natural studies, the study of nature, learned societies were construed to be those concerned with humanistic studies, that is to say, studies of man. Please take note of that meaning of humanistic, studies of man, in contradistinction to scientific, or studies of nature.

Soon after the founding of the Council there emerged a tendency to make a distinction among the learned societies concerned with the study of man between those categorized as "humanities" and those as "social sciences." Let me interject at this point that there is a certain sloppiness in this tendency to distinction just as there is in the distinction between the biological and physical sciences. At the founding of the Council in 1919 about half the original disciplinary societies would be construed later as humanities and half social sciences. All of them are disciplines concerned with reasoned efforts to present evidence for their findings about man as an individual and as a member of social groups, as a participant in a human fellowship. The social sciences such as economics, political science, sociology and psychology may be more disposed to search for categories, likes and unlikes, and to engage in methodologies of abstraction and reduction common in the natural sciences, but they also address important questions like the humanities for which such methods are inappropriate. There are important questions for which particular methodologies that have often been useful in natural science are not responsive to questions asked by social scientists and humanists. Within the incredible diversity of the universe around us our questions may lead to discoveries suggesting rules or laws like gravity, but we also encounter idiosyncratic phenomena like Napoleon and his career which call for understanding, and which often have consequences decades and even centuries later, including in our own times.

It was in the 1920s that there emerged in academe a tendency to divide humanistic studies, the study of man, into two broad categories: the humanities, in which the focus was mainly on the individual and his works; and the social, in which the focus was more on human social relationships. A reflection of this tendency was the establishment in 1923 of the Social Science Research Council. Even so, those disciplines that were called social sciences did not withdraw from participation in the ACLS. Further confusion was engendered in the 1950s by the rise of the designation "behavioral sciences." This name has not tended to displace in faculties of arts and sciences the earlier disciplinary divisions into humanities and social sciences, which accompany also divisions of physical and biological sciences. However, the designation "behavioral sciences" has acquired considerable currency in medical academic circles, even if the content thereof has not.

The story of the rise of "behavioral sciences" in academic parlance reveals that academic scholars in their ivory towers are not as far removed from the practical world as is commonly asserted. A bit of history is illuminating. In the fall of 1948 the trustees of the Ford Foundation, established by Henry and Edsel Ford, found themselves facing the need to undertake a greatly expanded program. While the Foundation had been established for the general purpose of advancing human welfare, the trustees felt the need for the Foundation's aims to be more specifically defined. The trustees therefore appointed an eight-man committee to prepare a report identifying more precisely program areas. The committee identified five program areas of critical importance for human welfare, the last of which was entitled "Individual Behavior and Human Relations."[3] The committee spoke to the need for more verified, more scientific, knowledge of human behavior on a wide front and the need for more support of research for the behavioral sciences—there is the word—and in particular for more support for pure research in the disciplines of psychology, sociology, and anthropology in contrast with applied research, the expenses of which were then more readily covered by other sources of funds. Henry Ford II, in the Fore-word to the trustees' Annual Report for 1951 stated that the trustees decided that the resources of the Foundation should be devoted to the five programs including, stated very succinctly, "the behavioral sciences."[4] The Foundation's 1952 Report fleshed out the meaning being given to so-called "behavioral sciences," which were to receive support, by saying that "techniques for the scientific study of the behavioral sciences need to be improved."[5] The flavor of what they meant was indicated by reference to support for a program "for the mathematical training of behavioral sciences." Particular reference was made to grants to psychologists, sociologists, anthropologists, economists, and to others "in the behavioral group." Is it any wonder that those individuals who would propose studies of human behavior cast in the abstract, reductionist quantitative methodology so common in the work of natural scientists, would present themselves as behavioral scientist applicants for the outpouring of largesse by the Ford Foundation? Overnight in the faculties of arts and sciences those social scientists who used numbers liberally in their research were willing to call themselves "behavioral scientists."

However, all was not peaceful on the campuses. The Ford Foundation's Report for 1953 stated (p. 64): "The Foundation's use of the term 'behavioral sciences' is not equivalent to the usual definitions of the social sciences as a certain group of academic disciplines." It added (p. 67):

> Of importance to the intellectual development of the behavioral sciences is the problem of improving their relationship with such disciplines as history, social and political philosophy, humanistic studies and certain phases of economics. Today this relationship is distinguished perhaps as much by recrimination and doctrinal dispute as by scholarly collaboration.[6]

Hence, the Foundation, in what might be called the beginning of a course correction, introduced a program of support for interdisciplinary research and studies. I can provide an illustration of the dispute to which the Foundation referred. When I went to Michigan as Dean of the College of Literature, Science, and the Arts (to use its early nineteenth century name), the chairman of the very large and active Department of Psychology was one of the most capable academic managers ever, Donald G. Marquis. He had been one of a group of social scientists on duty in Washington as World War II was drawing to a close and when the Pentagon found itself facing the probability of the need for a plan to integrate 11 million men in arms back into the economy and society at home. This was obviously a problem calling for substantial quantitative analysis to distinguish various kinds of groupings within the mass. Marquis carried this expertise with him when he became a member of the Ford Foundation committee and when he came to Michigan. As an entrepreneur for his department he was not loathe to present to the Ford Foundation his department as a behavioral science. On the campus, however, were others more wedded to the now traditional social science category, and who were resistant to the adoption of the label of behavioral science. In particular, James Kerr Pollock, chairman of Political Science, resisted this labeling, despite the fact that he had himself in earlier years used quantitative analysis with reference to studies of political parties in the United States, and indeed as chairman, he had actively recruited and supported some younger political scientists skilled in quantitative analyses of political phenomena. But he also believed in the importance of historical studies of political theory and in the analysis of the varied forms of government. Indeed, he had himself served as a political advisor to General Clay when the latter, after the surrender of Germany, had been the American viceroy over conquered Germany. In that role Pollock had been a principal drafter of the constitution of the Federal Republic of Germany. I well remember the day in the mid-1950s when I saw the President of Germany in the garden of Pollock's house place on the latter's chest the emblem of the highest honor which the Republic of Germany has to give in appreciation for his contribution to its government. Pollock simply did not like the narrowed connotations as to method which the behavioral science label had come to connote, and he did not want to neglect other equally important methods appropriate to his discipline.

I have taken your time for this little bit of history because of the addiction of medical men to the use of the behavioral science label. I well remember also the day in the mid-1960s when I left a meeting at the Shoreham Hotel and began walking over the bridge toward the center of Washington with Dr. Shannon of the National Institutes of Health. When he expressed an interest in expanding the boundaries of medicine to include attention to the behavioral sciences, I urged him instead to consider possible input into medicine more generally from the social sciences and humanities.

What a pity that the Ford Foundation fenced itself and its funds so narrowly. From 1954 through 1956 it continued providing research support explicitly for behavioral sciences. By 1957 it began offering its financial support for proposals in the humanities and arts. By then it had effectively contributed to the further divisiveness in the orientation among students of man and his culture. In any case, by the mid-1960s the phrase "behavioral and social sciences" had become common, the adjectives behavioral and social had become interchangeable. Researchers in the behavioral and social sciences commonly, though by no means exclusively, involved themselves in quantitative methodologies which made these fields seem more science-like. National Science Foundation support, hesitantly begun in the mid-1900s, was openly provided by the mid-1960s and in 1968 the NSF Act was amended specifically to include "social sciences."

By 1966 the long struggle to bring federal support to the humanities culminated in the establishment of the National Endowment for the Humanities, and the National Endowment for the Arts, though neither of these approximate the levels of support achieved for the sciences. These developments in funding relationships have not made any easier desirable collaboration among the various disciplines concerned with the study of man and his culture.

There is another problem of language which bedevils talk about medical education to which I should like to speak, in an effort for clarification in our subsequent discussions here. I refer to the variants of humanistic, humanities, humanism, humanitarian, humane. I have already referred to the use of humanistic as denoting those studies or disciplines which concern themselves with man, man as an individual and man as a social animal, what have now come generally to be called the humanities and the social sciences. My hope would be that this usage of humanistic, which is in the disciplinary world of the arts and sciences, would prevail.

Humanism is, as you will realize if you check Webster, an especially slippery word. It may mean devotion to the humanities. It may be used with an historical implication to refer to the cultural and intellectual movement which occurred during the Renaissance following the rediscovery of the literature, art, and civilizations of ancient Greece and Rome, and which stimulated a renewed interest in man and his capabilities. Related thereto is the use of humanism as a philosophy or attitude that is concerned with human beings, their achievements and interests; in this usage humanism is in contrast with deism, concern with God and his works or theology. Humanism may even be used to connote a dedication to human welfare. In our discussion here of education for the practice of medicine I suggest that we avoid the use of this slippery word humanism.

Variants with more relevance to our subject are humane, having the good qualities of human beings such as kindness, mercy or compassion, or humanitarian, concerned with the needs of mankind and the alleviation of human suffering. In medical literature those qualities regarded as desirable in physicians, values that should be expressed in physician behavior toward patients, are often described as humane or humanitarian. A similar expectation may be indicated by reference to a compassionate physician, one who shows empathy, a recognition by the physician of the suffering of the patient and an indication of his desire to give aid or support to the patient.

I assume that no one in his right mind would doubt the desirability of having physicians, professionals who undertake the healing and care of the sick, behave as persons who express in their lives, in their way of interaction with patients and their families, humane or humanitarian values or compassion. Physicians should be individuals who approach their patients with *attitudes* consistent with their samaritan function. It seems reasonable for those who admit applicants to medical schools or residencies to seek evidence of such values in applicants. Their further development in medical school might be encouraged by the provision of teachers who are themselves good role models of humane treatment of patients which trainees, medical students and residents, might seek to imitate.

But there is another aspect to this matter. The potential relationship of a physician, however humane or kindly may be his or her intent toward a patient, can be affected by the breadth and depth of his or her cognitive *knowledge* about human beings as whole operating individuals in human societies. A person with little knowledge and understanding of differences among human beings related to age, sex, race, education, class, occupation, and culture can approach others with the best of intentions, but can easily misunderstand, and be misunderstood by, others. Worse yet, there is a hazard for the compassionate physician in his approach to a suffering patient without a developed knowledge of himself and careful and informed reflection on the risks of transference and resulting distortions in understanding by him of himself and his patient. What is subsumed so lightly under the art of medicine itself has need of a scientific, an examined, cognitive underpinning, a base of rational knowledge about the diversities of human values and behaviors.

In addition to the development of an *attitude* appropriate to the role of a physician and the acquisition of *knowledge* about the diversity of human nature and the experience of man, the physician also needs to develop *behaviors, skills* in using himself or herself in personal relations with patients and their families, to acquire greater understanding of the patient's illness and/or disease. Humanists and social scientists have observed and thought about many of the actions and experiences of humankind; some of their ways of research and findings can be of assistance to physicians, as are some of the findings of physical and biological sciences with regard to the bodily aspect of man. The physician's acquisition of knowledge from the humanities, social sciences, and natural sciences does not make him a "professional" humanist or a social or natural scientist, with the motivations peculiar to scholars in the disciplines associated with these subject areas. The physician's purpose is rather to use all these sources of knowledge of man and nature as they contain information relevant to his role as a caretaker of the sick. In sum, then, the educational process required to educate a future physician for the biopsychosocial practice of medicine must embody a concern with the attitudes, knowledge, and skills or behavior of the candidate conducive to such practice.

There is clearly an established theory or view of what modern medicine is about, a *Weltanschauung* as the Germans would say, or perhaps, with apologies to Kuhn, a paradigm. It was referred to in the AAMC's GPEP Report as the Flexnerian form of medicine, the "specific benchmark against which all programs of medical education could be measured," the "form of medical education which has remained essentially unchanged for 70 years." This form obviously concentrates its attention on bioscientific diagnosis and treatment of diseased organs and tissues of the human body, as Flexner expressed it in 1910, the part of us that "belongs to the animal world."[7] For the present discussion, we will presume the continued acceptance of the Flexnerian form not as the whole but as part of a theory of medicine which embraces psychosocial aspects of illness which interact with the biological aspects. It will take, however, a conscientious effort for physicians to escape from the constricted view of Flexnerian medicine and to reach a broader concept of what should be involved in medical practice. As William J. Donnelly has described in a recent article, doctor talk itself reveals the confinement of medical thinking to a narrow view of a patient as a body only.[8] To accommodate a biopsychosocial view physicians will have to develop a richer, more varied language.

There is a cluster of ethical issues in medicine, the analysis of which may be furthered by the consideration of content from the humanities and social sciences, but to which I suggest we not devote special attention in this Conference, simply because there is now more recognition of their relevance to medicine than has yet been accorded these other, more neglected humanistic and social aspects of the business of medicine. Ethical issues may of course be raised in relation to matters under discussion.

Nor, I suggest, should this Conference include too much attention to disturbing pressures now confronting the medical profession. They have been poignantly expressed by a senior medical resident, Aran Ron, in a recent issue of the *American*

Journal of Medicine.[9] They have to do with external societal changes and pressures, financing arrangements and methods of cost containment, which have potentially deleterious impacts on doctor-patient relationships and the availability of health care for many people. Important as these external issues are, I suggest that we concentrate primarily on the immediate doctor-patient relationship. If doctors and patients between themselves cannot come to a better agreement about health care and the manner of medical practice desired, the chance for a better resolution of these societal problems is diminished thereby.

I wish to emphasize that *Dear Doctor*, the papers in this volume, discussions at Wickenburg and now our continuing discussions are not intended simply as contributions to a broader cultural background, grace notes if you will, for physicians, though they may incidentally contribute something to that end. They are intended rather as means to a better practice of medicine, to a better treatment of patients by doctors, perhaps even for a better life for practitioners of what can be a harrowing profession.

A hundred years ago there was in America what Dr. Kenneth M. Ludmerer has described as the "Innovative Period" in which physicians who had gone abroad primarily to German universities for training in biology were gathered together at Harvard, Johns Hopkins, Michigan, and Pennsylvania. It was their bioscientific curriculum that was articulated, and defended, by Flexner in 1910, and which was destined to become the standard curriculum for medical education in the twentieth century. At least three generations of physicians have been molded in that form. Bioscientific medicine rests on a hundred years of massive effort, none of which is rejected by those who argue for a biopsychosocial base for the practice of medicine. But the physician pioneers in psychosocial aspects of medicine that you will be hearing from, have hardly two decades of effort behind them. With attention now being given by some physicians to the psychosocial aspects of the patient, it would not be surprising if their more empirical exposure produced in the beginning useful insights, though recourse to communication with humanists and social scientists can lead them to more systematic research and to greater understanding of patients and their problems.

Medicine is a great and needed profession. It is in many ways a beleaguered profession. It seems unlikely that business as usual will be a sufficient response to the challenges facing it. What are the course changes that are needed?

REFERENCES

1. AAMC Project Summary Report. Physicians for the Twenty-First Century. *J Med Educ* 59:No.11, Pt. 2, 1984.

2. Odegaard, C. *Dear Doctor: A Personal Letter to a Physician.* Menlo Park, Henry J. Kaiser Family Foundation, 1986.

3. Ford Foundation. *Report of the Study for the Ford Foundation on Policy and Program.* Detroit, MI, 1949

4. Ford Foundation. *Annual Report for 1951.* Detroit, MI, 1951.

5. Ford Foundation. *Annual Report for 1952.* Detroit, MI, Ford Foundation, 1952.

6. Ford Foundation. *Annual Report for 1953.* Detroit, MI, 1953.

7. Flexner, A. *Medical Education in the United States and Canada.* New York, Carnegie Foundation for the Advancement of Teaching, 1910.

8. Donnelly, W.J. Medical Language as Symptom: Doctor Talk in Teaching Hospitals. *Persp Biol Med* 30:81-94, 1986.

9. Ron, A. The Perspective of Senior Medical Residents. *Am J Med* 82:302, 1987.

How Much Longer Must Medicine's Science Be Bound By a Seventeenth Century World View?

by

George L. Engel, M.D.

In any consideration of a scientific model for medicine that would qualify as a successor to the biomedical model, be it the biopsychosocial or any other, the fundamental issue is whether physicians can in their study and care of patients be scientists and work scientifically in the human domain. Or is medicine's human domain beyond the reach of science and the scientific method, an art, as the biomedical model in effect requires? How that question is answered depends on one's understanding of what is meant by science and the scientific method, and even more so on the form of the scientific paradigm that guides how knowledge is pursued and solutions to problems are sought. The fundamental distinction, we insist, is not between "science" and "art" but between thinking and proceeding scientifically and not so thinking and proceeding.

This is a question with which I found myself confronted very early in my life, in childhood actually, though obviously at so tender an age I was not yet aware that a problem existed and certainly not what the problem was. Let me explain. My two brothers and I were raised in the house of an uncle, Emanuel Libman (1872–1946), an eminent physician and scientist of the day. Our mother, who had undertaken to manage the household for her bachelor brother and widowed father, married late, and so it came to pass that in 1908 the Engel family became established in Libman's house, a four-story brownstone in mid-Manhattan, and that we three boys grew up in a setting dominated by Libman's professional activities. It was a scene of constant, at times frenetic, activity day and night. His office suite, including a library and laboratory, occupied the entry floor, the basement was a museum of pathology, his bedroom–sitting room, where he

113

often entertained visitors, was on the fourth floor, next to our own bedrooms. Libman's fame could hardly for long remain unknown to his nephews. All three of us soon enough found ourselves preoccupied with figuring out just what it was he did and why he was so famous and sought after. Not only did his patients number noted figures of the day, but visitors who came to the house to confer with him included the greats of medicine (and science) from all over the world, William Welch, Ludwig Aschoff, Alexis Carrel, Simon Flexner, Albert Einstein, on and on.

The family, of course, assumed we would in due course all become doctors, "like Uncle Manny." But Lewis (1909–1978) already by the time he was ten or eleven insisted otherwise. He would become a scientist, not a doctor. And indeed he did, singlemindedly devoting himself to chemistry, beginning with Chemcraft sets in a makeshift basement laboratory, his younger brothers serving as assistants. The bulk of his career was spent at the Harvard Medical School as an American Cancer Society Professor of Biological Chemistry and finally as chairman. My twin Frank (1913–1963) and I, however, vacillated. We read voraciously about science and scientists, medical and otherwise. Lew and his fellow graduate students in biochemistry teased us mercilessly for even considering so unscientific a life's work as that of a doctor. Yet here was Libman, renowned the world over as a clinician, possessed of extraordinary clinical skills and diagnostic acumen. But his scientific reputation rested not on that but on his work in the pathology and bacteriology laboratories. At the bedside he was the wizard, capable of astonishing diagnostic feats, at least according to family legend. In time I learned how often these were verified at post mortem, which at least lent to the family folklore a measure of credibility.

But why were these accomplishments with patients any less "scientific" than what he was doing in the laboratory? Frank and I used to puzzle over this together, but the answer eluded us. Both of us as early as 19 had begun working summers at the Marine Biological Laboratory at Woods Hole, Massachusetts. There we learned first-hand how to proceed scientifically in the laboratory.[1,2,3] There surely must be the answer, to exercise the same care to be accurate, thorough, reliable, relevant and comprehensible with patients as we had learned to do when working in the laboratory. And so we proceeded to do; and when we reached the clinical years, it paid off handsomely. Already by our fourth year at Hopkins, we both had earned the respect of our instructors for our not inconsiderable clinical skill and diagnostic acumen. Evidently Flexner's confidence in the laboratory as adequate preparation for a scientific approach at the bedside was sound after all.

And there the matter may have rested had it not happened, entirely by chance, that in 1941 I became involved in a research project on delirium with psychiatrist John Romano, the upshot of which was that I was over the next several years introduced not just to the human psychosocial dimensions of medicine, but even more importantly to what constituted the primary data of that realm and how to gain access thereto. The key proved to be a human relationship with dialogue the medium, and the interview, the scientific instrument for investigation of the human realm. Indeed, in my view, the interview is the most powerful, encompassing, sensitive and versatile instrument available to the physician and serves many different purposes. Yet none of us ever had any instruction in its use, much less in its underlying principles. From that time on my whole outlook, professional and scientific, was never again to be the same. The human dimensions of medicine had for me at last become accessible to scientific inquiry, just as had the heavens by the invention of the telescope. One could be scientific at the bedside after all!

To learn how this could be, we must first return to the question of what science is and what it means to be scientific. We begin with Charles Odegaard's definition:

SCIENCE

Science represents man's most persistent effort to extend and organize knowledge by reasoned efforts that ultimately depend on evidence that can be consensually validited.[4]

Note that this definition places no limits on what phenomena may be the subject of scientific inquiry.

SCIENCE

The scientific method is complete in the sense that there do not exist phenomena in nature which, in principle, cannot be examined by application of the scientific method of valid data accumulation and verification.[5]

Advances in science depend on developing means and techniques of inquiry that are appropriate for the phenomena under investigation and the conditions and circumstances under which such can be studied. Viruses are not to be studied with the naked eye at absolute zero. By the same token scientific study of human phenomena requires human means and human circumstances.

What is meant by scientific "paradigm" or "model"?

PARADIGMS

Paradigms are constituted from the concepts, assumptions and rules that guide workers in their pursuit of knowledge and the solution of problems in a given field.

Paradigms gain status to the extent that they are successful in solving problems, and they lose status as paradoxes multiply.[6]

Paradigms powerfully influence what scientists select to study and how they go about doing so. The paradigm acts subtly both as a value judgment and as a motivator to proceed in one way or another. Scientists are not necessarily fully aware of the paradigm they are using and how it may influence their judgments and motivation. Paradigms that become part of the scientist's cultural background risk becoming dogma. Kuhn captures the power of paradigms in the following:

PARADIGMS

The proponents of competing paradigms . . . see different things when they look from the same point in the same direction. . . . what cannot even be demonstrated to one group of scientists may seem intuitively obvious to another.[6]

This statement exemplifies the conflict confronted by medicine over the past three centuries. While hardly anyone can dispute the extent to which medicine is "concerned with all the various aspects of man's humanness," as Rene Dubos so aptly put it,[7] medicine's adherence to a seventeenth century paradigm predicated on the mechanism, reductionism, determinism, and dualism of Newton and Descartes automatically excludes what is distinctively human from the realm of science and the scientific.

The seventeenth century paradigm is a system of thought in which scientists as objective observers are to regard nature as independent from themselves and unaffected by their act of observation. Developed as an approach to nature as it surrounds man, such a paradigm provides no means to accommodate human processes, and never was intended to. In medicine this has become entrenched in the biomedical view that what is human about medicine and its practice constitutes but an art. Accordingly, the physician has come to be seen as operating scientifically and medicine judged to be properly scientific only when dealing with bodily processes, not when dealing with patients as people.

Yet for almost a century the classical model of physics on which such a way of thinking is based has increasingly been undermined. In the course of the development of relativity theory and quantum mechanics, physics has been obliged to reintroduce the human being into the scientific equation.[8-11] Pure objectivity and total detachment of the investigator from his material no longer constitute inviolable criteria for what is to be accepted as science or scientific, not even ideally. The influence of the investigator has become a factor to be reckoned with, not one that can ever be completely corrected for. Thus relativity theory was formulated around the notion of an observer, while quantum mechanics promoted the observer to a participator who in the very process of investigating affects the outcome of his observations. The scientist and the object of his investigation, it turns out, are not separable precisely because every observational act in itself embodies an element of subjectivity, namely, the observer's decisions as to what to observe and how.[8] The new physics not only shatters the illusion of the scientist as totally detached, it also documents the interconnectedness and interdependence of all levels of organization of natural systems.

The fundamental contrast between the seventeenth and twentieth century paradigms goes well beyond the old philosophic controversy between "realism" and "idealism." Though derivative from experimental studies in physics, the twentieth century paradigm in fact establishes the indispensability of including what is human in the explanatory system; it acknowledges that science is a human activity and that what the scientist does cannot be separated from what is being inquired into. Let us contrast the seventeenth and twentieth century paradigms in a schematized and obviously oversimplified way:

THE SEVENTEENTH CENTURY PARADIGM
(Newton, Descartes)

What is being studied exists external to and independent of the scientist, who discovers and characterizes its properties and behavior.

This is the essence of the objectivity that is required if one is to be considered a scientist.

Nobelist chemist Marie Curie early in this century left no doubt what she considered to be the scope of science. "Science deals with things not people," she bluntly put it.[12] And of course she was correct. The science she knew never was intended to encompass human affairs—and it doesn't! That is precisely the issue confronting medicine and which medicine has yet to face.

In contrast, let us consider the changes in our understanding of science wrought in the twentieth century.

THE TWENTIETH CENTURY PARADIGM
(Einstein, Heisenberg)

What is being studied is inseparable from the scientist, who devises mental constructs of his/her experiences with it as a means of characterizing his/her understanding of its properties and behavior.[8]

In this view scientists are not studying a world external to themselves but rather those particular interactions taking place at the moment between themselves and the phenomena in question and under whatever conditions they are being studied. Heisenberg put it: "What we observe is not nature itself, but the interplay between nature and ourselves; science describes nature as exposed to our way of questioning."[13]

Delbruck acknowledged the irony of this discovery:

THE TWENTIETH CENTURY PARADIGM
(Einstein, Heisenberg)

The observational act is a unitary deed of which our choice is an active subjective component. . . . in the drama of existence we play the dual role of actor and observer! How bizarre . . . that this realization, . . . so antithetical to the conceptual foundations of science, should be forced upon us by atomic physics.[8]

Actually this is nothing new for clinicians working with patients. We have always been aware of the difficulty of defining objectively what we are learning from our patients and of doing so independently of the subjective means we employ for our observations. Rather than dismissing such an approach as outside of science, it now appears that the same limitation holds for all of science; it does not constitute a criterion whereby the scientific is to be differentiated from the nonscientific.

Seen from this perspective, the clinical encounter, which defines the conditions and setting in which scientific work with patients proceeds, constitutes not an obstacle to objectivity, but rather another mode of data collection, one the consistency and reliability of which can be perfected once it is recognized wherein the scientific study of one person by another differs from the study of nonhuman material or phenomena. In the latter, be the material an enzyme, organ, or an experimental animal, it is acted on and reacts to the investigator but itself can neither initiate nor control the process of investigation, much less give an account thereof. The human subject can do all of these and in so doing not only becomes an active participator in his own study, but also provides access to an inner world of experience not possible in lower forms of life. Accordingly, in the clinical setting the scientific effort actually becomes a joint undertaking to be negotiated between physician and patient (or surrogate), one which requires the physician as scientist to be operating concurrently in two modes, one observational, the other relational.

The two modes address quite different categories of data and with different criteria. The observational mode is suited for phenomena that can be observed with the senses (or extensions thereof), e.g., the color of the skin, manifest behavior, the heart rate, or the level of serum bilirubin. These are the classical data of empirico-analytic inquiry, often capable of precise mensuration as well as accurate description, which, if necessary, can be ascertained without the patient's active participation.

In contrast, a relational mode is required to deal with data in the uniquely human realm of articulated language, symbols, thoughts and feelings by means of which what we privately experience is organized and communicated and relationships established and managed. In this mode dialogue serves to clarify the meaning and verify the information that is being reported.[14] It is through dialogue that the physician learns the nature and history of the patient's experiences and clarifies on the one hand what they mean for the patient, and on the other, what they might mean in terms of other systems of the natural hierarchy, be they biochemical and physiological, or psychological and social. This is the process of clinical reasoning. It is a mode in which clarification of meaning and of establishment of veracity take precedence over measurement.

By tradition the observational mode, as represented by the empirico-analytic approach, is accorded scientific status, while the relational mode, as dialogue, is not. Yet in clinical practice the physician always operates in both modes at the same time, making observations while engaging in dialogue and vice versa. The two processes thus not only are complementary and supplementary with respect to the results achieved, they are also interdependent in operation. Information being obtained in one mode may not be accessible in the other but may be clarified, elaborated, verified, or refuted by access to the other mode, sometimes simultaneously. Anxiety verbally denied may be verified by demonstrating tachycardia and cold sweaty hands. The meaning of "OK" in response to "How are you?" may be questioned if a gesture of helplessness is observed to accompany it. A patient's report of "palpitation" may be elaborated through direct examination or electronic recordings. Accordingly, the two modes constitute not alternative, but a single integrated means for data disclosure, clarification and interpretation in the clinical realm. Rather than a combination of one scientific and one non-scientific (or unscientific) approach, they represent a single approach that has evolved logically out of the historical fact that inquiry into the nature of illness and patienthood has always had to depend both on what the patient can communicate verbally and nonverbally and on what the physician can observe.[15–18] Only the constraints of the classical seventeenth century paradigm exclude the relational from the category of the scientific, as Marie Curie so bluntly informed us.[12]

Dialogue is in fact the only means whereby the patient can acquaint the physician with those inner experiences which had led him to consider himself ill in the first place, and therefore to solicit medical help. By the same token dialogue enables the physician to reconstruct with the patient a plausible sequence of events ("history") from which hypotheses may be developed, which in turn may be explored by further dialogue as well as by other means. As every clinician well knows, the reasoning process (clinical reasoning) proceeds actively and concurrently with the data-collecting procedures of observation and dialogue, not seriatim as more commonly is the case with laboratory experiments. As an integral component of the process whereby the clinician gains knowledge of the patient's condition, it is thus clear that *dialogue is truly foundational to scientific work in the clinical realm.*

Once the foundational character of dialogue is acknowledged, the essential complementarity of the human and the scientific premised by the twentieth century paradigm becomes apparent. This is inherent in the fact that dialogue as a means of data collection and processing is itself regulated by conditions that determine human relationships. Accordingly, completeness and accuracy of the data are correspondingly enhanced by optimizing those human circumstances which are most likely to facilitate dialogue. The physician has no alternative but to behave in a humane and empathic manner, that is, to understand and be understanding, if the patient is to be enabled to report clearly and fully. Only then can the physician proceed scientifically; to be humane and empathic is not merely a prescription for compassion, as medical educators would like us to believe; it is a requirement for scientific work in the clinical realm.

Biomedicine's rejection of dialogue as a genuinely scientific means of data collection is evident in the neglect of instruction and supervision in interviewing, not to mention in clinical data collection altogether, and in the preference for the case presentation as a method of clinical teaching, one in which students may display their ability to organize and discuss findings, but not reveal the methods and skills whereby they had come by the data in the first place, least of all their interpersonal engagement with the patient.[19–23] Such pervasive inattention to the conditions and requirements for reliable data collection in itself constitutes nothing less than an antiscientific attitude.

The paradox is apparent. While all would agree, physician and patient alike, that the judgments, decisions and recommendations made by physicians as far as possible should be based on demonstrated scientific principles and on evidence, that is, on data that are accurate, complete, and obtained through methods of demonstrated reliability, reliance on the seventeenth century paradigm excludes from that requirement information that is only accessible through the medium of human exchange, and that on the grounds that it is "subjective" and by inference thereby "inherently unreliable." In a current journal appears a typical example of dialogue bypassed in favor of direct recourse to diagnostic procedures. The following are direct quotations, but the emphasis is added:

LIQUEUR LUNG

. . . We describe a condition—"liqueur lung"—in which hemoptysis was produced by the aspiration of Bucca. . . .

A 22-year-old healthy nonsmoking man presented after coughing up a cup of bright-red blood. *The initial history and physical examination were unrevealing.* A chest roentgenogram, arterial blood gas levels, the complete blood count, indexes of coagulation, the platelet count, and the blood urea nitrogen concentration were all normal.

Bronchoscopy with a flexible fiberoptic instrument was performed within 24 hours, since the hemoptysis totaled 75 ml of blood. The trachea and right mainstem bronchus were erythematous and friable and contained a small quantity of fresh blood. No infectious organisms or neoplastic cells were found in the tracheobronchial specimens submitted for analysis. *The bronchoscopic findings, prompted additional questioning of the patient.* He revealed that he had experienced a coughing paroxysm the previous evening. He had been at a party and had "guzzled from a bottle of Bucca." While drinking in this manner he began to choke and cough repeatedly. A few hours later, frank hemoptysis began.[24]

"The initial history [was] unrevealing"! There may have been some unusual extenuating circumstance accounting for the failure to learn of the aspiration on first contact with this man, but in my experience it is more likely accounted for by the physician's low valuation of what patients have to report coupled with lack of skill to elicit information in the first place.

Similar disregard for the applicability of a scientific approach is revealed by the resident who upon coming to the bedside of a new patient in the emergency department immediately requested the three visitors clustering around the bed to leave.* Queried on what she had based such a decision, she could only respond that such was customary; at least so she had been led to believe by her mentors. She had never before seriously considered systematically examining its rationale. In that realm her

---

*In my teaching rounds how the student or resident engages with the patient is an integral and indispensable part of the exercise. To facilitate that process, we do not rely on the usual case presentation method. The person who knows the patient acts as a resource, responding to questions, but not otherwise participating. The rest of the group, including the faculty member, are to know nothing in advance about the patient. The exercise begins with one member demonstrating for all of us how he/she initiates and pursues for five to ten minutes contact with a patient totally unknown and being seen for the first time.[21]

otherwise well-practiced "inquiring and scientific mind" simply was not operative.[25]

And what about the medical grand rounds patient applauded by the audience for his good fortune at having been in the emergency department rather than still on the street when his cardiac arrest occurred? Only the medical student, whose earlier tape-recorded interview I listened to, had learned how tremendously upset the man had become when the housestaff, failing in their effort to insert an arterial line, had left him alone in the cubicle; the arrest occurred a few minutes later.[26] At the rounds it was the student who voiced curiosity about the possibility of a connection between the man's emotional state and the arrest; no one else did.[27] Here an "inquiring scientific mind" was at work, and that because this student had a scientific model in mind which facilitated his access to the data from which such a question could logically be framed.

To appreciate relationship and dialogue as requirements for scientific study in the clinical setting highlights the natural confluence of the human and the scientific in the clinical encounter itself. It is not just that science is a human activity, it is also that the interpersonal engagement required in the clinical realm rests on complementary and basic human needs, especially the *need to know and understand* and *the need to feel known and understood*. The first, to know and understand, obviously is a dimension of being scientific; the second, to feel known and understood, is a dimension of caring and being cared for. Both may be seen as derivative and emergent from biological processes critical for survival in the phylogenetic as well as ontogenetic senses. The need to know and understand originates in the regulatory and self-organizing capabilities of all living organisms to process information from an everchanging environment in order to assure growth, development, self-regulation, adjustment, and survival.[28] In turn, the need to feel known and understood originates, in man at least, in the transition from the biological mutuality of intrauterine life to the social mutuality of neonatal life that inaugurates the corresponding life-long need to feel socially connected with other humans. In the course of development fulfillment of both needs comes in a complementary fashion to equate with a personal sense of confidence, security, and belonging. The need to know and to understand ultimately achieves its most advanced development in the disciplined curiosity that characterizes scientific thinking. The need to feel known and understood manifests itself in the continuity of human relationships and in the social complementarity between perceived helplessness and the urge to help. Herein then converge the scientific and the caring (samaritan, pastoral) roles of the physician.

Falling ill typically involves for the patient a disruption in that unique continuity of knowing and understanding and of feeling known and understood that ordinarily characterizes health and well being. Typically a patient comes for help because he is experiencing something strange, different, discomforting, or disabling which he does not understand and/or does not know how or feel able to handle by himself. At the same time he believes— or hopes—the doctor does understand and does know how to handle the situation. The largest part of what the patient feels disturbed by is known only to himself and will remain so unless and until communicated. Two considerations loom large in the patient's decision to share such information and to entrust himself and his care to a physician. The first is confidence that the physician is competent; the second is the expectation, or at least the hope, that the physician will be understanding and that he, the patient, will feel understood. Thereby is the patient motivated to relinquish autonomy and share privacy, often to a degree greater than may be true of almost any other human relationship.

For the patient, to feel understood by the physician means more than just feeling that the physician understands intellectually, that is, "comprehends," what the patient is reporting and what may be wrong, critical as these are for the physician's scientific task.[29] Every bit as important is it that the physician display understanding about the patient as a person, as a fellow human being, and about what he is experiencing and what the circumstances of his life are. "Do my doctors know who I am, who I have been, who I still want to be? Do they understand

125

what I am going through, my suffering, my pain, my distress? Do they understand my hopes and aspirations, my fears and shames, my vulnerabilities and strengths, my needs and obligations and my values? Above all, do they sense my personhood and my individuality? Do they acknowledge my humanity? Do they care?"

The physician's need to know and understand at first glance may seem more exclusively cognitive. But while scientific understanding does mean getting all the facts and getting them straight, every bit as important is for the physician to display that human understanding which is so necessary if the patient is to feel understood. Again, the two are complementary. For when expression of human understanding on the part of the physician is not forthcoming and the patient does not feel understood, then trust and confidence may be impaired and with it the patient's capacity and willingness to collaborate—critical if the physician's scientific aims are to be accomplished.

Let me illustrate these principles with an experience I once had as a visiting professor asked to conduct a medical grand rounds. My aim was to demonstrate the requirements for a scientific approach to a patient with and about whom I had no prior relationship or knowledge. The setting was a large amphitheatre on the stage of which I was to work with the patient.

The patient, a man in his mid-forties, arrived in a wheelchair. After an introduction by the resident, I first asked whether the exercise had been explained to him. He at once angrily complained that not only had no one explained the exercise, he had been left unattended in a cold drafty corridor outside the auditorium; altogether no one seemed to care what happened to him. To my awkward efforts at commiseration and apology, he broke eye contact and turned away. He shrugged indifferently when I asked if he would be willing to tell the doctors something about the illness. My "How have you been feeling?" evoked a sarcastic "How would you feel?" We were already at an impasse.

For me to establish my role with him as samaritan, to say nothing of my role as scientist, would require us first somehow to touch one another's individuality, to meet each other as fellow beings. As the physician, the task was mine, not his, and the instrumentality would be dialogue. Only through the give and take of dialogue could we begin to take a measure of each other. Under the circumstances in which we found ourselves, inquiry about his illness seemed the most appropriate entree, awkward as that was.

And as I had anticipated, his initial responses were laconic and limited to symptoms; he said virtually nothing about himself. To try to broaden our engagement beyond those narrow confines, I repeatedly interjected into his bare symptom reporting such questions as, "Where were you when that happened?" "What were you doing?" "Who else was there?" Bit by bit he began to add a few personal details. Then, quite unexpectedly one particular item caught my attention. A vegetable garden! It was while tending a vegetable garden that he first developed chest pain. Here at last was something uniquely personal. Surely having a vegetable garden in the midst of the squalor and congestion of the urban ghetto where he lived must say something of the man behind the angry facade. My curiosity and surprise were genuine, and he must have felt it, for he at once responded to my echoing query, "You were gardening?" with a willingness to elaborate until then not evident. In surprisingly few minutes quite another human being began to emerge, a man with a life story all his own.

Now I was getting to know a former migrant field worker who had successfully established himself as an auto worker in Detroit, only to lose his job in the recession after almost a dozen years of steady employment. Health insurance lapsed, savings melted away, his home and car were repossessed, and his wife and his children finally went back South to her parents' farm. He remained behind still hoping for re-employment, living alone in a rooming house. The garden he had scratched out of the rubble of a vacant lot was one last effort to sustain his image of himself as self-sufficient and responsible. Falling ill and being hospitalized in a large public hospital was the last blow.

As this story began to emerge, we all moved closer, the patient and I and the grand rounds audience, drawn together by shared feelings, despair and concern, pride and admiration, anger and frustration, until all was silence but for the patient's now soft but engaging voice and my occasional sound or word of concern or encouragement. Finally he fell silent, his head lowered, eye contact broken, the upper lid line angled, his eyes moist, his hands resting motionless on his thighs. I knew he was close to tears. Hardly aware of it, I had already pulled my chair closer to his. I placed my hand on his and, squeezing it gently, said softly, "It's been a tough time for you, hasn't it?" At once tears formed. Still silent, he wiped them away with the tissue I had offered him. Then with a faintly apologetic smile, he raised and let fall his hand in the gesture of helplessness, adding "What else could I do?" I nodded and said nothing. Nothing needed to be said. We both now knew we understood each other. After but a brief pause we resumed the exploration of his illness. In short order, I could be confident that I had all the pertinent facts about his illness and about himself and his circumstances to justify the presumptive diagnosis of myocardial infarction and to consider plans for his further study and care. Most of all mutual confidence and trust had been established between us. Yet our total acquaintanceship had spanned but eighteen minutes. When I reluctantly brought the interview to a close, we shook hands. This time it was he who squeezed my hand. "Thank you, doctor," he said, though surely he knew we would never meet again.

In this example the requirement to be human in order to be scientific is evident at many levels. In my role as scientist merely the exercise of an inquiring scientific mind would not be enough. I had also to make possible the conditions without which my inquiring scientific mind could not have access to the material required for my task, that is, I had to promote a productive dialogue. To gain access I had also to establish myself in the samaritan role. Through behavior alone I had to achieve in a few minutes, and with a complete stranger, and a hostile one at that, the mutuality of understanding necessary if one person is to entrust life and well-being to another. But my ability to do so was not merely a matter of intuition, common sense and experience, important as these may be. Quite to the contrary, it rested on a body of knowledge and a set of principles about human behavior and relationships arrived at through systematic inquiry, that is, scientifically.

To illustrate such application of scientific thinking in the human domain, let us focus on the two or three minutes which culminated in the patient's crying. During the first minutes of our meeting, he hardly impressed me as a man likely to cry. But once he began his litany of losses and frustrations, crying became not just a possibility, but a possibility the risks and benefits of which I had to weigh. On the one hand, crying and being comforted by me could facilitate my goal of engendering a feeling of understanding between us; on the other, it might evoke shame and embarrassment, even anger and loss of control, especially for this man in the public glare of teaching rounds. In addition, I also had to keep in mind possible medical contraindications to crying, as might occur had the patient just had eye surgery, for example. Thus even the task of establishing myself in the samaritan role itself called for a scientific approach. It would not do for me simply to rely on my own impulses or intuitions. My judgment as to whether I should encourage or inhibit his crying had to be based on evidence reliably elicited and on knowledge and principles scientifically arrived at; not only that, the decision had to be reached while a choice was still possible. How did I do so?

First, while actively engaging in dialogue, I was at the same time monitoring the likelihood of his crying. This I did by paying attention to signs known to presage crying, such as facial expressions (e.g., angling of the upper lid), gestures (e.g., helplessness), body movements and positions (e.g., sagging of his shoulders), behaviors (e.g., bringing a finger to his eye), and what he was having to say and how (e.g., sad content, a "catch" in his voice).[30–35] *Second*, I watched and listened for indications of physical and emotional movement toward or away from me, as sustaining or breaking eye contact, inclining his body toward or away from me, or sharing or withholding intimacies. *Third*, I noted his responses to my behavior, as when I moved closer, spoke more softly, or indicated sympathy with his plight. All of these each of us knows more or less intuitively, but we are not necessarily aware that we know, or what it is we know, which informs us that crying may be imminent. Here the scientific process involves examining and analyzing the intuitive, establishing its validity through means the reliability of which can be assayed and deriving principles the generalizability of which can be tested by other means and/or by other investigators.

Einstein once characterized science as "nothing more than a refinement of everyday thinking."[36] Wherein was my approach here any more scientific than how I might have behaved in everyday life? What is perhaps most obvious is that not only was I prepared in my mind for the possibility that the patient might cry—patients do cry, after all, even those least expected to—I also had an agenda covering what issues might need to be addressed in his case were crying to loom as a possibility; and I had a design in mind for how to do so.

Further, from information derived from scientific study I had learned reliable signs whereby to monitor with minimal, even subliminal, attention to the prospects of his crying. Such cognitive monitoring is one of the refinements Einstein alluded to, namely the establishment and use of uniform and agreed upon criteria to identify and characterize natural phenomena. By recourse to such a taxonomy of crying, in addition to my own intuitive sensitivity,[31] I was able to track this man's progress toward crying at the same time I was processing the data which would determine whether I should try to encourage him to cry or whether I should try to forestall it, also a process for which criteria exist. In so proceeding, I remained fully conscious of and deliberately attentive to the collaborative nature of my work with the patient; I was not simply being a cold, detached observer of another's distress. Nor was I distracted from our overall agenda by the necessity to address his distress. On the contrary, I used my human inclination to assuage distress as a means to forge ties with the patient and to engender thereby the mutual understanding required for the patient and me together to pursue our emerging scientific agenda.

We have defined science in its broadest historical sense as man's most persistent effort to extend and organize knowledge by reasoned efforts that ultimately depend on evidence that can be consensually validated.[4, 37, 38] Note that this characterization of science—and scientific—is independent of any particular paradigm. Paradigms by their very nature serve to create a frame of mind receptive to answering some questions and sanctioning certain methods while discouraging and ruling out others. Often operating as silent assumptions taken fully for granted, we have seen how in medicine adherence to the seventeenth century paradigm of physics has in the clinical realm actually engendered attitudes that are antiscientific and behaviors that are unscientific. Science and being scientific have increasingly come to be defined in terms of that paradigm. As a result, the human realm either has been excluded from accessibility to scientific inquiry or the scientific approach to human phenomena has been required to conform to the reductionistic, mechanistic, dualistic predicates of the biomedical paradigm. To do so constitutes misapplication of that paradigm.[39] What the advocates of the universality of the biomedical model have failed to appreciate is that, like its seventeenth century counterpart in classical physics, the biomedical model represents a limiting case the utility of which is in no way diminished as long as its use is restricted to the phenomena for which it was designed. The biomedical model needs no defense, neither with respect to its past accomplishments nor to its future utility, as long as that rule is applied. But to do otherwise is to be *unscientific*; to advocate doing otherwise is to promote dogma and become *antiscientific*. To become more fully scientific, medicine requires a paradigm capable of encompassing the human domain. The twentieth century paradigm of physics assumes the human dimension as a given for all scientific endeavor and in that sense eliminates an obstacle to paradigm development in medicine. As Einstein poetically expressed it, the relationship of the successor paradigm, whether called systems or biopsychosocial, with its predecessor, the biomedical, depends on accepting the latter's limitations:

THE LIMITING CASE

Creating a new theory (paradigm) is not like destroying an old barn and erecting a skyscraper in its place. It is rather like climbing a mountain, gaining new and wider views, . . . but the point from which we started

131

out still exists and can be seen, although it appears smaller and forms a tiny part of our broad view gained . . . on our way up.

From the new theory it is clear in which cases classical physics is valid and wherein its limitations lie.[40]

Conclusions

1. The biomedical model, like the model of classical physics, represents a limiting case; it cannot be used as a criterion for science (or "scientific") in medicine.

2. Application of the biomedical model outside its limits is unscientific; advocacy of such application promotes dogma and is antiscientific.

3. Scientific medicine requires a paradigm capable of encompassing the human domain. The twentieth century paradigm of physics assumes the human dimension as a given for all scientific endeavor and hence meets that requirement for paradigm development in medicine.

4. The general systems theory derived biopsychosocial model and the more fully articulated infomedical model of Foss and Rothenberg are promising candidates for successor paradigms to the biomedical model.[26, 41–45]

REFERENCES

1. Engel, G. L. and I. Chao. The comparative distribution of organic phosphorus compounds in the cardiac and striated muscles of limulus polyphemus. *J Biol Chem* 108: 389–393, 1935.

2. Engel, G. L. and R. W. Gerard. The phosphorus metabolism of invertebrate nerve. *J Biol Chem* 112: 379–392, 1935.

3. Webster, M. D., F. L. Engel, E. P. Lang, W. R. Amberson. The influence of pH upon the elimination of hemoglobin by the perfused frog's kidney. *J Cell Comp Physiol* 5: 399–412, 1934.

4. Odegaard, C. E. *Dear Doctor. A Personal Letter to a Physician.* Menlo Park, Henry J. Kaiser Family Foundation, 1986.

5. Zimmerman, D. W. A note on the completeness of the scientific method. *Psycholog Record* 34: 175–179, 1984.

6. Kuhn, T. S. *The Structure of Scientific Revolutions,* 2nd Ed. Chicago, University of Chicago Press, 1970.

7. Dubos, R. Hippocrates in modern dress. *Proc Inst Med.* Chicago 25: 242–251, 1965.

8. Delbruck, M. *Mind from Matter? An Essay on Evolutionary Epistemology.* Palo Alto, Blackwell Scientific Publ., 1986, p. 289.

9. Comfort, A. On physics and biology. Getting our act together. *Perspect Biol Med* 29: 1–9, 1985.

10. Bernstein, J. John Archibald Wheeler. *Johns Hopkins Magazine* 37: (5) 23–33, 1985.

11. Morowitz, H. J. Myasthenia gravis and arrows of fortune. *Hosp Practice* 21: (3) 179–192, 1986.

12. Curie, M. cited by J. Goodfield. Humanity in science: A perspective and a plea. *Science* 198: 580–585, 1977.

13. Heisenberg, W. *Physics and Philosophy, The Revolution in Modern Science.* New York, Harper, 1958, p. 81.

14. Wiggins, O. P. and M. A. Schwartz. Techniques and persons. Habermasean reflections on medical ethics. *Human Studies* 9:365–377, 1986.

15. Engel, G. L. Clinical observation. The neglected basic method of medicine. *JAMA* 192: 842–852, 1965.

16. Engel, G. L. Enduring attributes of medicine relevant to the education of the physician. *Ann Int Med* 78: 587–593, 1973.

17. Engel, G. L. Commentary on Schwartz & Wiggins: Sci-

ence, humanism and the nature of medical practice. *Perspect Biol Med* 28: 362–365, 1985.

18. Reiser, S. J. *Medicine and the Reign of Technology.* Cambridge, Cambridge University Press, 1978.

19. Reichsman, F., F. E. Browning, J. R. Hinshaw. Observation of undergraduate clinical teaching in action. *J Med Educ* 39: 147–163, 1964.

20. Payson, H. E. and J. D. Barchas. A time study of medical teaching rounds. *New Engl J Med* 273: 1468–1471, 1965.

21. Engel, G. L. Some limitations of the case presentation method for clinical teaching. An alternative approach. *New Engl J Med* 284: 20–24, 1971.

22. Engel, G. L. Are medical schools neglecting clinical skills? *JAMA* 236: 861–863, 1976.

23. Shankel, S. W. and E. L. Mazzaferri. Teaching the resident in internal medicine. Present practices and suggestions for the future. *JAMA* 256: 725–729, 1986.

24. Conetta, R., F. M. Tamarin, D. Wogalter, R. D. Brandstetter. Liqueur lung. *New Engl J Med* 316: 348–49, 1987.

25. Engel, G. L. Physician-scientists and scientific physicians: Resolving the humanism-science dichotomy. *Am J Med* 82: 107–111, 1987.

26. Engel, G. L. The clinical application of the biopsychosocial model. *Amer J Psychiat* 137: 535–544, 1980.

27. Engel, G. L. Sudden and rapid death during psychological stress. Folklore or folk wisdom? *Ann Int Med* 74: 771–782, 1971.

28. Riedl, R. *Biology and Knowledge. The Evolutionary Bases of Reason.* New York, John Wiley & Sons, 1984.

29. Evans, D. A., M. R. Block, E. R. Steinberg, A. M. Pen-

rose. Frames and heuristics in doctor-patient discourse. *Soc Sci Med* 22: 1027–1034, 1986.

30. Engel, G. L. The care of the patient: Art or science? *Johns Hopkins Med J* 140: 222–232, 1977.

31. Engel, G. L. Signs of giving up, in *The Patient, Death and the Family*, S. B. Troup and W. A. Greene, Eds. New York, Charles Scribner's Sons, 1974, pp. 43–69.

32. Darwin, C. *The Expression of the Emotions in Man and Animals* (1872). New York, D. Appleton, 1896.

33. Schmale, A. H. Needs, gratifications and the vicissitudes of the self-representation. A developmental concept of psychic object relationships. *Psychoanal Study Society* 2: 9–41, 1962.

34. Schmale, A. H., D. Tinling, L. Eby. Experimental induction of affects. *Acta Med Psychosom* 1: 1–8, 1967.

35. Engel, G. L. Grief and grieving. *Am J Nursing* 64: 93–98, 1964.

36. Einstein, A. *Out of My Later Years*. New York, Philosophical Library, 1950, p. 59.

37. Flexner, A. *Medical Education. A Comparative Study*. New York, MacMillan, 1925.

38. Harrison, A. S. Common elements and interconnections. *Science* 224: 939–942, 1984.

39. Engel, G. L. Misapplication of a scientific paradigm. *Integrative Psychiat* 3: 9–11, 1985.

40. Einstein, A. and L. Infeld. *The Evolution of Physics*. New York, Simon and Schuster, 1938, p. 159.

41. Brody, H. The systems view of man: Implications for medicine, science and ethics. *Perspect Biol Med* 17: 71–92, 1978.

42. Engel, G. L. The need for a new medical model: A challenge for biomedicine. *Science* 196: 129–136, 1977.

43. Engel, G. L. The biopsychosocial model and the education of health professionals. *Ann NY Acad Sci* 310: 169–181, 1978.

44. Schwartz, M. A. and O. P. Wiggins. Systems and the structuring of meaning: Contributions to a biopsychosocial medicine. *Am J Psychiat* 143: 1213–1221, 1986.

45. Foss, L. and K. Rothenberg. *The Second Medical Revolution. From Biomedicine to Infomedicine*. Shambhala, Boston, New Science Library, 1987.

Scientific and Humanistic Medicine:
A Theory of Clinical Methods

by

Michael Alan Schwartz, M. D. & Osborne P. Wiggins, Ph. D.

Science vs. Humanism—Crisis in Present Day Medicine

Does humanistic medicine have a future? Is it even possible to practice humanistic medicine in an area marked by an explosive growth of medical knowledge and technology? As medical science makes rapid strides and as the old forms of health care are replaced by newer, apparently less personal forms, humanistic medical practice grows ever more problematic. Increasingly, there seems to be a conflict between humanistic and scientific medicine. While everyone might lament the loss of the humane physician, the longing for such a caretaker appears more and more to reflect nostalgia and wishful thinking.

Against this tide, efforts have recently been made to promote humanism in medical education. For example, the American Board of Internal Medicine has required "high standards of humanistic behavior in the professional lives of every certifiable candidate," and other Boards have declared their resolve to follow the lead of the internists.[1] In addition, the Board of Internal Medicine and the Society for Research and Education in Primary Care Internal Medicine have developed guides for educators and physicians to encourage humanistic attitudes and behaviors among doctors.[1,2]

A backlash to such efforts has already surfaced, however. Following a three-year study supported by the Association of American Medical Colleges, the Panel on the General Professional Education of the Physician and College Preparation for Medicine issued a report, the *GPEP Report*, which along with many other recommendations referred briefly to humanistic concerns in medicine.[3] The suggestions in this report were quite tentative, possibly even "equivocal," focusing more on how to teach than on what to teach.[4] Nonetheless, the rather limited recommendations of the *GPEP Report* were received quite suspiciously. Although a *Commentary on the GPEP Report* by a Working Group appointed by the Council of Deans (COD) and the Council of Academic Societies (CAS) cleared the *GPEP Report* of charges that it would contribute to "lessening the relative importance of scientific education (p. 347),"[5] the COD-CAS group did state that "medical education must always project a balance between the scientific and the humanitarian aspects of medicine (p. 347)."[5] Furthermore, according to the COD-CAS group, many basic and clinical scientists believed that the GPEP panel failed to recognize the problem of "the loading of additional courses into the preclinical phase" of medical education (p. 349).[5] While the nature of these courses went unspecified, most new courses added over the past decade have had a humanistic or social scientific content.[4]

But why would anyone worry about the possibility that humanism in medical schools would lead to "lessening the relative importance of scientific education?" The concern would seem to arise only if humanism and science were wholly different. Humanism, in other words, is assumed to be non-scientific. Only such an assumption would lead one to seek ways to "project a balance between the scientific and the humanitarian aspects of medicine."

Furthermore, if there is indeed a dichotomy between medical science and medical humanism, then humanism is surely doomed. For the forces that have edged humanism out of medicine in the past will only grow more potent in the future. Technology, specialization, the mass of scientific facts, and the cost of medical science will continue to increase. If these realities are truly the obstacles to humanism, appeals for humanism—although they will inevitably sound more and more enticing—also will sound more quixotic. If humanism is to be reinstated in medicine, then, it cannot be at the price of abandoning the highest commitment to scientific practice.

But is the dichotomy between scientific and humanistic medicine a valid one?[6,7] Is humanism by its very nature non-scientific? Perhaps most efforts to heal the breach between scientific and humanistic medicine have failed so far because they have, with notable exceptions,[7-15] uncritically accepted this assumption. In this essay, we intend to re-examine the nature of scientific activity in order to show that physicians can be truly scientific *only* if they are also fully humanistic. Showing this, we shall argue that genuine science and genuine humanism in medicine, far from remaining irreconcilable, in fact require one another.

Before we begin this re-examination, however, we would like to sketch the nature of the historical forces which have led people to assume that science differs so greatly from humanism. To these historical forces we shall apply the names "the spirit of abstraction" and "the fallacy of misplaced concreteness."

THE DICHOTOMY BETWEEN SCIENCE AND HUMANISM

Scientific concepts and theories can be developed only by abstracting from the features of things that we experience in everyday, prescientific life. Scientific concepts are developed precisely by "abstracting from. . . ." That is, we disregard or set aside certain properties of things in order to focus on other properties of them. Such abstractions permit precision and exactitude and thereby facilitate clarity in conceptualizing and theorizing. But the more precise a concept, the more features of things it must ignore or exclude.[16]

In a previous paper we have described the pervasive tendency in modern culture to approach reality *solely* from abstract points of view and to forget that such abstractions have excluded other aspects of reality. Following Gabriel Marcel, we have called this modern tendency "the spirit of abstraction."[17] Those features of things which our abstract concepts capture are then taken to be the *basic* features of things. As a result, all other properties of things are denigrated to a secondary status: they are deemed "merely subjective." And the abstract features, now seen as basic, come to be viewed as alone disclosing the true, fundamental nature of things. But what is taken to be "truth" is merely a segment of reality, an abstractly reduced portion of a whole. The spirit of abstraction consists in forgetting that these parts are mere parts so that partial truths are mistaken for the whole.

Present-day science with its powerful mathematico-logical formulations provides highly abstract points of view on reality. We inherit these theories in a ready-made form through our education and culture, and we thus tend to overlook their immense abstractness. In this manner, these theories are falsely identified as the "concrete truth" of reality. And, as a consequence, the truly concrete world—the world of everyday experience—is ignored and denigrated as illusory, subjective, and shallow. The assumption that abstract perspectives alone can penetrate to the basic nature of things has been called "the fallacy of misplaced concreteness."[18] In fact, abstract and concrete perspectives are both objective and real. Furthermore, abstract perspectives are developed out of the more basic concrete ones, not the other way around. The spirit of abstraction, however, falsifies our view of the world by leaving us blind to the more concrete—and equally real—properties of things.[16,19]

Let us examine an example. A biomedical scientist might equate peptic ulcer disease with an ulcer crater in the duodenum and with various aberrant complex pathophysiological and hormonal processes. Such a scientific description of peptic ulcer disease sets aside the patient's complaints in order to focus on structural and physico-chemical realities. Because of the spirit of abstraction and the fallacy of misplaced concreteness, these complaints are denigrated to a much less important rank in order to focus on the pathology and pathophysiology of the illness. Biomedical practitioners tend to assume that these characteristic difficulties alone constitute the "truth" or "objective reality" of disease.[8,20] If physicians restrict themselves exclusively to such an abstract view of the illness, the other qualities tend to be lost from sight.

Richard Baron provides us with a telling illustration of the error of this line of reasoning.[21] He refers to several studies on ulcer treatment which all demonstrated that the anatomic fact of an ulcer cannot be correlated with patients' complaints. In one major study, for example, after four weeks of treatment, 55 percent of patients whose ulcers were unhealed were asymptomatic, regardless of treatment group. In addition, 27 percent of patients whose ulcer had healed endoscopically continued to have ulcer symptoms.[22] This study has been duplicated,[23] and it has been cited in a recent review which questions the value of the current medical treatment for ulcers.[24] Moreover, a recent review of the use of diagnostic procedures in gastrointestinal (GI) hemorrhage recommends "early endoscopy especially in upper GI bleeding, if the gastrointestinal lumen can be cleared of blood"[25] despite the citation in this same review that two prospective randomized controlled studies showed no benefit from this approach.[26,27] In such a situation, Baron comments:

> Our attachment to the anatomicopathologic fact of the ulcer persists despite solid clinical evidence that "seeing" the ulcer does not change the clinical outcome. Clearly, we are fascinated with disembodied anatomic realities, even when we have substantial reason to believe that they relate less and less to what bothers our patients or what ultimately happens to our patients (p. 607).[21]

Baron further maintains that our understanding of disease has progressively moved away from the patient towards a reification of a model of disease. To view the disease as simply the ulcer cra- ter and its associated pathophysiology is to mistake an abstract part of the illness for the whole. Thus the spirit of abstraction governs the biomedical definition of the problem. "Our under- standing of the nature of the disease," Baron claims, "is limited by (the biomedical) model, and entire aspects of the phenome- non of illness remain inaccessible or incomprehensible to us (p. 607)."[21] Moreover, since illnesses such as irritable bowel syn- drome or hiatus hernia presently lack anatomicopathological facts, many physicians tend to take the complaints and suffering of patients with such illnesses much less seriously.

Patients with even vaguer complaints and non-localizable le- sions are relegated by biomedical reductionism to a netherworld of hypochondriacs and malcontents. There is, so they are told, nothing "medically" wrong with them. Whatever is wrong with them is seen as falling outside of the purview of scientific medicine.

The fact that modern science develops and utilizes abstrac- tions need not lead to this shortsighted view, however. The spirit of abstraction and the fallacy of misplaced concreteness are not necessary logical consequences of scientific abstraction. They arise for historical rather than logical reasons; but nevertheless, this spirit and this fallacy do tend to influence our times.[4,19] The marvelous technological powers that issue from scientific abstractions in medicine are certainly impressive. Such abstractions are misused, however, when they are seen as our sole access to reality. What must be opposed, consequently, is the spirit of abstraction. For such a narrow spirit prevents medical practitioners from becoming not only fully humanistic but also fully scientific. The spirit of abstraction leads us to dismiss much of the directly given data. It restricts scientific evidence to that which falls under our more abstract concepts and theories. This restriction ignores other evidence: it ignores the evidence that is directly given in our more concrete experience and thought. Doctors fail to be truly scientific as long as they ignore this more concrete evidence: they fail to consider all the evidence regarding illness and health. In order to take this more concrete evidence into account, we must regain our appreciation of that more concrete mode of human experience that necessarily precedes the high-level abstractions of modern-day science.

We shall attempt now to sketch the main features of this more concrete kind of experience. We shall do so in order to show how science emerges from it. At that point we shall be able to demonstrate how scientists can approach this more concrete domain in order to take its evidence into account. In this way physicians will be able to achieve a more complete *scientific* understanding of patients and also have a more *humanistic* appreciation of them.

THE LIFEWORLD AND THE LIVED BODY

Following Edmund Husserl, we give the name "lifeworld" to the world as we experience it in its concrete fullness, prior to viewing it through the abstractions of science.[19,6,28] The lifeworld, in other words, is the world as we encounter it in our everyday, prescientific experience. In the lifeworld we encounter other people, cultural objects, and natural things with all of their concretely given properties. Thus, these people, objects, and things have for us the features they have in our prescientific, everyday experience, not those properties that scientific abstractions attribute to them.

For example, apples, as we encounter them in the lifeworld, are red and sweet; they are not objects with particular molecular and chemical characteristics. As another example, the bodies of other people, as we experience them in the prescientific lifeworld, are not the organisms of which biologists or physiologists speak. The body of my neighbor as he waves to me from across the street is a meaningful and expressive reality. Through his bodily actions he expresses his feelings and his intentions, and he communicates them to me.[12] And in understanding his greeting, I do not distinguish between its "physical" parts and its "mental" parts: I do not apprehend his bodily movements as "the physical" and the intentions expressed by such movements as "the mental" parts. I rather apprehend his greeting as an indivisible unit. My understanding of him is "psychophysically neutral": it makes no distinction between his mind and his body.[6] The same holds for my experience of my own lived body. If I respond to my neighbor by smiling and waving back, I do not distinguish between one part of my smile, the kinesthetic sensations involved in moving my lips, as the physical component and another part, the emotion of friendliness, as the mental part. My experience of my own lived body is psychophysically neutral.

The organism that biologists describe through their abstract concepts is not this meaningful, expressive, and communicative lived body. Biologists, in order to characterize the organism, must abstract from its concrete meaningfulness and expressiveness. Let us call this meaningful and communicative human body of prescientific experience the "lived body," and let us distinguish it terminologically from the "organism" that is abstractly depicted by biologists and physiologists.[28]

Understanding and Communication in Everyday Life

In my prescientific experience I can understand my neighbor's feelings, ideas, choices, and purposes as he expresses them through his words and behavior. And he can understand me. Let us call this ability to comprehend the feelings, ideas, decisions, and intentions of another person "understanding."[29,30] Understanding, then, is our access to other people as concrete wholes. It is the way in which we apprehend other people and their experiences apart from any abstract concepts developed by scientists. As thus defined, understanding is crucial to the communication and interactions that pervade everyday life.[31]

Understanding another person through communication is always a matter of degree. When my neighbor waves to me, I need to understand him to only a very limited extent in order to grasp that he is merely signaling "hello." At the gasoline station the pump reads $16, and I hand the attendant a $20 bill. Without saying a word he hands me $4 and I drive away. Our interlocking intentions, silently expressed in deed and gesture, have been communicated sufficiently for our purposes at hand. This communicative understanding guides and informs our transaction.[32] Therefore, the practical activities of daily social life could not take place without such mutual understanding. Furthermore, the goals of these practical activities circumscribe the extent to which we need to communicate with one another.

Sometimes we need to understand one another to relatively great extents. Especially in intimate relationships but also in many other instances I need to grasp large portions of another person's experience in significant detail. Thus I come to understand how this other person experiences his or her world. For example, I may come to understand how my friend feels about his work, his love and concern for his family, and his hopes, expectations, and fears for the future. I know my friend well enough to understand his motives and behavior in especially complex situations. Suppose that I am with him when he suddenly falls ill. Knowing his values and personality, I understand his reluctance to seek treatment. I understand, although he does not tell me—and perhaps does not even know himself—that out of a sense of responsibility toward his family and his job he cannot face being ill at this time. Moreover, my understanding of him may enable me, by appealing to values that I know he holds, to persuade him to seek medical help despite his initial reluctance.

In this way our mutual understanding informs our communicative interaction. And furthermore, our communication alters, deepens, and extends our understanding of one another.[32]

TYPIFICATIONS AS SKILLS IN EVERYDAY LIFE

This communicative understanding of people along with my perception of things is always informed by certain typifications.[33,31,34,35] When I see my neighbor waving his hand, I typify this piece of behavior as a friendly greeting. Moreover, when I drive my car through a new part of town, I typify the objects going past me as cars and trucks. Such typifications are not explicit acts of conceptualization; they rather occur at a pre-conceptual, purely perceptual level of everyday experience. I do not *conceive* the objects moving past me *as* cars; I rather immediately *see* them *as* cars. Typification is "seeing as . . ." or "understanding as. . . ."[36] When I sit down at my desk in the morning, I need not explicitly scrutinize all of the objects on my desk in order then to recognize what they are. Typifications occur automatically and with greater immediacy. As I sit down at my desk, I immediately see some of the things as books, others as letters, and even others as pens.

Because typifications are pre-conceptual activities, they can be viewed as "skills" as defined by the biologist, Michael Polanyi. Polanyi characterizes a skill as follows:

> the aim of a skillful performance is achieved by the observance of a set of rules which are not known as such to the person following them (p. 49).[37]

When I perceive an object moving past me as a car, I do not do so because I explicitly compare features of that object with a set of rules that define cars. I do not know "the set of rules" that I am using when I immediately typify the object as a car. I simply and immediately see the object as a car. Much the same can be said about riding a bicycle. If I have mastered the skill of riding a bicycle, I do not explicitly observe a "set of rules" as I thoughtlessly ride my bicycle down the road.

The Taken-For-Grantedness of Everyday Life

The typifications that inform our everyday experience are pervaded by a certain taken-for-grantedness.[31] For example, in my everyday life I simply take it for granted that the man across the street who appears to be my neighbor is in fact my neighbor and that the waving of his hand expresses a greeting to me. I could, of course, doubt that he is my neighbor or that his hand waving indicates a friendly greeting. But in my ordinary life I usually harbor few such doubts. Or consider another example. In my prescientific life I simply assume that my friend feels well unless something in his behavior or appearance prompts me to think otherwise. If he looks like I am accustomed to him looking, I merely take it for granted that he feels well. I assume, in other words, that things truly are what they appear to be. I take the appearances of things for granted; I do not persistently question, doubt, or suspect them. I may come to doubt these appearances, however, if something occurs which is unexpected or is inconsistent with them. I assume that my friend is well until he enters my home looking run down, glassy-eyed, and red-nosed. His directly given appearance then shatters my taken-for-grantedness and compels me to ask about his health. Only this unexpected counter-evidence can challenge my assumption that he is well and force me to doubt it.

From Prescientific Life to Scientific Activity

Scientists will avoid precisely this taken-for-grantedness of prescientific experience. They will adopt instead a critical attitude toward whatever appears to be the case. The critical attitude can guide us in our scientific investigations of concrete realities. This attitude can also guide us in the use of the typifications that we learn to apply as scientists. And, finally, the critical attitude of science can also lead to the development of concepts and theories that are more and more abstract. We must now examine these features of scientific activity in some detail.

SCIENTIFIC ACTIVITY: THE CRITICAL ATTITUDE AND THE SEARCH FOR EVIDENCE

Scientific activity, we maintain, is any human activity that rigorously adopts "a critical attitude."[38] As scientists we circumvent the taken-for-grantedness of everyday life. In the critical attitude required by science, I do not need counter-evidence to compel me to doubt that things are what they appear to be. As a scientist I am rather *persistently doubting* that things truly are what they appear to be. The scientific attitude is a sustained suspiciousness and uncertainty of what appears to be the case. And because I remain steadily suspicious and doubtful, I seek evidence to decide what things truly are. But when evidence emerges, I remain critical even of the significance of this evidence. And consequently, I seek more and more evidence to help me make my decision. The scientific attitude requires, therefore, that I seek as much evidence as I can possibly obtain regarding the phenomena in question.[38] As a result, the critical attitude of the scientist always includes a *tentativeness* or *provisionality* regarding any claim to knowledge. No scientific belief is simply "true." Every scientific claim is only tentatively or provisionally true, pending the gathering of further evidence regarding it.

SCIENTIFIC TYPIFICATIONS AND IDEAL TYPES

Because of his or her critical attitude, the scientist applies concepts, theories, or techniques to people and things only tentatively and provisionally.[38] This holds as well for the typifications that the scientist uses.[31] Through work in his or her field, the scientist progressively acquires the skills of typification peculiar to that field. For instance, the medical scientist can identify, often at a glance, the emphysematous patient by perceiving his quite characteristic "barrel chest." Of course, this medical typification must function within a critical attitude: although this person *looks like* a victim of emphysema, he may not in truth be one. The barrel chest may be a result of skeletal changes associated with aging in patients who are asymptomatic and exhibit none of the physiological findings of pulmonary emphysema. Or a patient may have emphysema and not have a barrel chest. Because of these alternative possibilities, scientific typifications—however automatically and immediately they may occur—must be used critically. Moreover, they must be applied provisionally and tentatively, always pending the gathering of further evidence. Nonetheless, typifications can initiate and guide fruitful scientific inquiry.

Moreover, manifold aspects of the patient's life are typified by the physician. The doctor typifies, for example, the patient's personality style (such as "hysteric" or "passive-dependent"), socio-cultural background (such as "elderly ethnic lady"), or value system (such as "solid citizen" or "bohemian"). Initial impressions about diagnoses can follow from typifications, but so can initial ways of talking to patients as well as initial impressions about what an illness may mean to a patient.

While typifications are preconceptual, the features apprehended through those typifications can always be explicitly conceptualized.[34] Such explicitly articulated concepts are called "ideal types."[39,40] For instance, a physician may be able to typify a barrel chested person as emphysemic. But this typical barrel chestedness can then be included with other features in the definition of the syndrome of emphysema. This syndrome—expressly conceived as a constellation of signs, symptoms, pathophysiology, course, and outcome—is an ideal type. Such conceptualization of syndromes are called "ideal" because they specify features which are sometimes found in real cases but sometimes are not: not all emphysemic people exhibit the characteristic barrel chest. It is frequently overlooked, however, that the concepts which spell out syndromes are based upon typifications and are thus based upon preconceptual skills for *seeing* people *as* barrel chested, breathless, etc.

SCIENTIFIC UNDERSTANDING AND COMMUNICATION

Any aspect of life becomes "scientific" as long as it is examined with a critical attitude. Accordingly, those features of people which are available to us through understanding and communication, namely, their ideas, feelings, and intentions, could be critically investigated.[30,32,41] Within such an attitude we would remain firmly suspicious and doubtful toward what appears to be a person's ideas, emotions, or purposes. Thus we search for evidence regarding these realities. We would speak with him or her and thereby elicit further information and evidence regarding the person's experience. We would closely scrutinize the person's facial expressions, body gestures and posture, vocal intonations, behavior, and what he or she says. These pieces of evidence, of course, would have to be examined within the context of the person's culture and society: a particular gesture or expression in one culture might convey a feeling quite different from that which the same gesture or expression would signify in a different culture. And moreover, these different data would have to be carefully compared with one another. For example, the person who tells me he is feeling fine but whose facial expression exhibits distress has directly presented me with data that seem to contradict one another and that therefore require supplementation through more evidence. As a result, I might ask him certain questions or make certain statements in order to elicit a particular response from him. His response may then evoke even further questions from me as I attempt to ascertain precisely what he is experiencing. In this way I am attempting to interact with the person and thereby understand his or her emotions, conceptions, and intentions. But I am attempting to understand them *scientifically*: I am thoughtfully examining the direct evidence that would verify or falsify my belief that the person has one intention rather than another, that he or she feels one way rather than some other way, etc. This communicative understanding is *scientific* because it moves beyond the taken-for-granted attitude of our everyday understanding of people's experience and behavior and adopts a critical attitude toward them. We submit that such scientific communicative interaction should play as much a role in medical practice as laboratory tests and procedures.

Scientific communicative interaction must draw, however, upon the understanding of people we have already acquired through our interactions with them in everyday life. Thus our prescientific experience in the lifeworld serves as the basis for all scientific work. Suppose, for instance, that a patient reports that she is "having trouble sleeping." I know what she means because I am familiar with the experience of "having trouble sleeping" through my everyday life with others. Of course, this prescientific familiarity, acquired through my participation in the lifeworld, receives further definition and precision from the scientific notion of "insomnia." And with my more scientific knowledge of insomnia, I can initiate further scientific investigations regarding its cause: I might consider various possibilities, including an acute situational reaction, sleeping pill abuse, an affective disorder, or a rarer organic cause such as sleep apnea. But these scientific conceptions would themselves make no initial sense to me if I did not first have some more direct knowledge of sleeplessness and its effects. The scientific must always draw upon the prescientific, however far it develops beyond it.

The extent to which we need to understand another person scientifically is always a matter of degree. And this degree is delimited by our purposes at hand. I may need to understand a patient's system of values in detail in order to persuade him to take his medicine. Or I may be able to succeed in this task with only a very limited understanding of him. It may take considerable communicative interaction with my patient in order to appreciate his sense of self, including how he believes he is seen by other people, and thereby to convince him to wear a much needed hearing aid.

Of course, my understanding of my patient may be mistaken. Even after much effort has been spent in communicative interaction, I may conclude that he refuses to wear the hearing aid because of vanity regarding his fashionable appearance. But my understanding may be erroneous. In fact, he cares little for fashion. He rather refuses to wear the hearing aid because he does not want to appear weak. Why did I make this mistake? Let us suppose that I made it because I myself am extremely conscious of fashion and I assume that everyone is. I have erroneously projected onto him my own concerns regarding appearance.

The possibility of such mistakes in our efforts to understand other people has led critics to denigrate all understanding as subjective and unscientific. But this possibility of mistakes simply shows that understanding is like any other mode of human experience: we can always make mistakes. Our mistaken beliefs could always lead us to "project" our own presuppositions onto other people and things. There is no talisman to protect human experience from error other than the critical attitude and its demand for more and more directly given evidence.

We would like to emphasize the possibility that as a result of the process of communicative interaction either partner may change his or her views. For instance, in speaking with my patient about the need for him to wear a hearing aid, I may learn something about him such that I finally conclude that it would be better for him to use the device only on particular occasions. Or he may finally come to see, although he had not wanted to recognize it earlier, that in fact he should wear the hearing aid.

THE SCIENTIFIC ATTITUDE AND THE LIVED BODY

Above we introduced the notion of the "lived body" and contrasted it with the abstract scientific conception of the "organism." The lived body is the human body as we experience it in everyday life: it is that body through which people act on things and express their feelings, ideas, and intentions.[28,42]

Now we can abandon the taken-for-grantedness within which we usually encounter the bodies of other people and adopt a critical attitude toward them. Within this critical attitude we can undertake a scientific examination of them. We would like to stress the fact that by simply adopting a critical attitude toward the lived body, we do not necessarily transform it into and begin to conceive it as an organism. Even within the critical attitude of science the body we see remains the meaningful, expressive, and communicative lived body. We have now simply altered our attitude toward it. When I encounter a patient with a blank, expressionless face and a body devoid of much movement, I, as a medical scientist employing a critical attitude, remain uncertain and doubtful of this apparent blandness. I carefully look for further evidence. Perhaps this person is in fact extremely casual and emotionless. But my doubting raises other possibilities. Perhaps this is the flat affect of a major mental illness. Perhaps this paucity of expressiveness reflects a neurological disease such as Parkinson's disease.

The lived body is the human body in its concrete fullness, prior to those abstractions regarding it which capture only precisely selected portions of it.[28] But because of this concrete fullness of the lived body, we may interpret it in a variety of different ways. The bland and expressionless face of my patient could be interpreted as issuing from an anxious reaction to the medical encounter; it could arise from simple fatigue; it could result from the illnesses mentioned above and also be exaggerated by anxiety or fatigue. Of course, with the acquisition of more evidence regarding this patient, some or even most of these possible interpretations may be falsified. But there will always be ambiguity: the blandness may reflect anxiety, not from the medical encounter, but from some personal, social, or economic predicament. Through interaction with the patient the doctor may elicit evidence that discloses this predicament, or he or she may not. But even if the physician does elicit such evidence, ambiguity remains: the patient may have some deep, underlying complex that produces anxiety in a situation that does not ordinarily call for anxiety. And there are even other issues that remain ambiguous: if the patient is indeed anxious, why does he have a blank facial expression rather than a fearful or an agitated one?

In contrast to the precision and exactitude attainable at the higher levels of abstract concepts, this ambiguity embedded in concrete human reality might appear scientifically hopeless. But the fact that the evidence of concrete reality is ambiguous is simply that, an ascertainable *fact*. And scientific activity consists in the careful examination of facts. Science is rigorous fidelity to the evidence. If the concrete data are inherently ambiguous, scientists must confront this evidential ambiguity in its own right, without trying to avoid its reality.[30,28,43] In contrast to what many people assume, precision and exactitude are not essential requirements of science. Faithfulness to the evidence within the critical attitude is the essential requirement of scientific activity. If the evidence is ambiguous, this ambiguity must be scientifically respected. In fact, forcing ambiguous evidence into exact and precise formulations for the sake of some presumed "science" distorts this evidence and thus violates the fundamental requirement of genuine science. We like to call this error of forcing all evidence into exact and even mathematical molds the "Procrustes Complex," in recognition of the mythological figure who, in his own bloody fashion, first demanded precision at all costs.

But even with regard to ambiguous evidence, not just any interpretation is acceptable. The evidence rules out some interpretations as false while it confirms others to varying degrees.[38] Thus within the critical attitude the medical scientist can come to deem certain interpretations more likely or better confirmed than others while he or she considers other interpretations less likely or probably false. As the evidence grows, certain interpretations take on greater prominence and likelihood. In short, all interpretations stand or fall by the degree to which they conform to the directly given data.

Karl Jaspers' Laws of Understanding

The physician and philosopher Karl Jaspers has most clearly addressed this problem of the ambiguity of concrete evidence. Jaspers formulated six laws to guide such scientific understanding.[30] He developed these laws for psychiatric practice in particular, but they apply to all scientific investigations involving a doctor–patient relationship.[41,44]

1. *Empirical understanding is an interpretation.* Jaspers' first law of scientific understanding arises from the fact that this understanding is *scientific*, i.e., it operates within a critical attitude and thus requires as much evidence as possible for its conclusions. As Jaspers himself formulates this demand for evidence, "Every step in understanding is . . . linked to objective phenomena" (p. 356).[30] Because of this strict requirement for evidence, no claim for understanding achieves absolute certainty. Each claim always stands in need of further testing by comparing it with more directly given data. We can say, therefore, that the claims of understanding remain *hypothetical*: they remain tentative, pending

further evidence. Jaspers calls such hypothetical claims "interpretations."

2. *Understanding opens up unlimited interpretations.* Jaspers, as we have said, recognizes the ambiguity of the concrete data of understanding. And from this recognition he draws the inference that the same data are subject to many different interpretations. The multiplicity of such interpretations does not betoken arbitrariness, however. For each interpretation must be able to verify itself through reference to evidence. Therefore, Jaspers concludes "as empirically accessible material grows, understanding becomes more decisive" (p. 359).[30]

3. *Understanding moves in a deepening spiral.* This ambiguity, in Jaspers' view, can be reduced by a circular movement from a particular fact to the whole and then from the whole back to the part. For example, a person's emotional withdrawal in the face of a rebuff makes sense to us, but this meaning remains limited and nonspecific. But within the context of a larger understanding of the person's life and situation, this withdrawal can acquire for us a more specific and concrete meaning. And with this more specific interpretation of the part, we can return to the whole once again and make greater sense of the person's life and situation.

4. *Opposites are equally meaningful.* Opposing interpretations can be based on the same evidence. For example, we can understand the stoicism of a patient as stemming from bravery and nobility. But we can also understand this same stoicism as motivated by profound fears and a complete inability to face up to a difficult predicament. Thus when only fragments of evidence are available for interpretation, we must remain deeply suspicious of our own conclusions. We should always search for other ways of interpreting the evidence. Otherwise we may be settling for an a priori interpretation that could mislead us by predisposing us to notice only the evidence that conforms to a precipitous conclusion.

5. *Understanding is inconclusive.* Understanding a person's feelings, ideas, and intentions has its limits. Jaspers mentions two such limits. First, a person's feelings, ideas, and intentions are

rooted in neurophysiological processes that can be explained but not understood. Second, human freedom makes it impossible to understand fully and completely the motives at work in generating emotions, ideas, and purposes.

6. *To understand is to illuminate and expose.* Understanding unearths negative and positive aspects of the patient's life. Such understanding can expose a person's weaknesses and faults, but at the same time it can also disclose his or her strengths and potentialities. For physicians who so often get "behind the scenes" during particularly difficult times in their patients' lives, this final law of Jaspers issues a warning against the debunking cynicism that can emerge from a busy practice.

Scientific Explanation

Scientific activity can take on a more abstract form, however.[45,46] We can abstract from or disregard human ideas, emotions, values, and purposes. Indeed, we can abstract from the mental components of life altogether. Having performed such abstractions, we can focus exclusively on mechanisms and causal processes. Events are then treated as causal mechanisms and as, therefore, subsumable under general causal and perhaps even mathematizable laws. The laws of glucose metabolism or dose response curves of medications exemplify such accounts. Let us call these abstract causal accounts "law-governed explanations."[30,47]

Sciences, such as biology and physiology, have developed a highly abstract conception of the living organism.[16,48] From this abstract point of view the organism is conceived as a machine: a system of interdependent causal mechanisms whose extremely complex structure serves highly differentiated functions. When the organism is conceived in this manner, we can develop law-governed explanations to account for its operations in health and in illness. Although this point of view is abstract, it is also, we wish to emphasize, an important way to comprehend *real* features of the body. Obviously, such a conception of the organism as a law-governed machine has a powerful and most beneficial payoff for medical practice.

This abstract notion of the organism can be developed, however, only by setting aside other properties of the body. It disregards, for instance, the expressiveness and meaningfulness of the lived body. A full scientific account of the body, we maintain, must include both the body as machine and the lived body as expressive and communicative reality.[28]

Traditional biomedicine with its premium on law-governed explanations has tended to ignore the lived body and focus exclusively on the organism.[6,49,50] From this perspective only law-governed accounts of the organism are deemed truly scientific. But this conception of medical science, we repeat, is unduly restrictive. It limits medical science to explanations of the organism through mechanistic and mathematical laws.

Phenomena of health and illness which can be subjected to law-governed explanations, such as the organism as machine, can be defined only by abstracting extensively from manifold properties of human life. But with this abstraction much is gained: in the ideal case it permits us to quantify the law-like explanations that we employ. And with mathematical explanations comes the power to predict and even control outcomes.[48]

Such power to predict and control outcomes with mathematical precision is extremely attractive to a practical science like medicine. Thus the temptation arises to maintain that medical practice should strive for mathematical explanations of all of the conditions of health and illness so that these conditions can be effectively controlled. Biomedicine succumbs to this temptation. Biomedicine reduces all of medical understanding to such law-governed explanation. But this temptation is to be resisted if some of the factors that contribute to health and illness cannot be subjected to mathematical explanations. And indeed some of these factors by their very nature seem to elude measurement and mechanistic explanation. Of course, one can never foresee which of these factors can be mathematized and explained. But because mathematization can occur only through an abstraction that sets aside manifold properties of things, those properties abstractly set aside would still resist mathematical explanation.

And these non-mathematizable factors may nevertheless contribute to health and illness.[6]

THE HIERARCHY OF THE SCIENCES

Scientific activity is based on the lifeworld. But such activity
must relinquish the taken-for-grantedness of everyday experience in the lifeworld and begin to examine phenomena from
within a critical attitude. Within this attitude both concrete and
abstract realities can be scientifically investigated. Consequently, we can arrange the various sciences in a hierarchy in
terms of the degree of concreteness and abstractness of the realities that comprise them.[6,16,19]

This hierarchy, however, sets forth a hierarchy of the *pure* sciences. That is, scientists in these fields seek only the *truth* of their
chosen subject matter. They seek "knowledge for its own sake."
All practical goals or purposes remain extraneous to these pure
disciplines.

Such pure sciences are to be contrasted with the practical sciences. The activities of practical scientists are delineated by the
practical goals or *aims* that they strive to achieve. Practical scientists appropriate knowledge attained by pure scientists and use
this knowledge in the service of their own goals.[6]

MEDICINE AS A PRACTICAL SCIENCE

Medicine is a practical, not a pure, science. Physicians do not
seek knowledge of illness and health for the sake of this knowledge alone. They rather seek this knowledge in order to use it in
order to further the practical goals of medicine: the promotion
of health and the amelioration of illness in patients. Any facts,
theories, concepts, techniques, or procedures of the pure sciences may be used by physicians if they can serve these goals.
And aspects of the pure sciences that cannot serve these practical
goals remain irrelevant to medicine. Physicians, like other practical scientists, can pick and choose from all of the pure sciences
knowledge or techniques that are relevant to promoting health
and ameliorating illness.

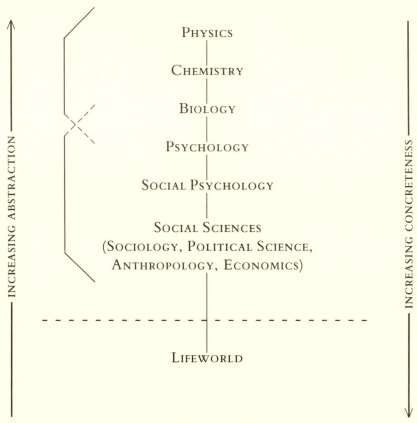

INCREASING ABSTRACTION

INCREASING CONCRETENESS

PHYSICS

CHEMISTRY

BIOLOGY

PSYCHOLOGY

SOCIAL PSYCHOLOGY

SOCIAL SCIENCES
(SOCIOLOGY, POLITICAL SCIENCE,
ANTHROPOLOGY, ECONOMICS)

LIFEWORLD

The Hierarchy of the Pure Sciences

Because medical practitioners can move among the many pure sciences and use components of any of them, medical science has no definite place in the hierarchy of the pure sciences that we have diagrammed above. Physicians draw freely on many sciences—both pure and practical ones—without needing to identify themselves with any specifiable group of sciences. Moreover, because patients are human beings, doctors may utilize components of the humanities and the arts, such as philosophy, literature, and religion. And yet because of their special goals of promoting health and ameliorating illness, physicians must go beyond what other fields provide and develop concepts and techniques that directly serve their goals. Thus concepts and techniques arise that are peculiar to medicine. For example, the disease of emphysema is a concept peculiar to medical science. While our present-day understanding of emphysema is quite sophisticated, no such understanding could have arisen without drawing on pure sciences such as anatomy, physiology, and physics. Moreover, devices used to diagnose and manage emphysema draw on knowledge and techniques gained from practical sciences such as engineering. Emphysema is not a concept in these other sciences, however. This concept becomes formulated only when we begin to focus on the goals of the promotion of health and the amelioration of illness.

Doctors with their practical aims thus utilize a wide-ranging assortment of approaches, concepts, and techniques which originate in other disciplines. As a consequence, medicine appears to possess no unity, and doctors seem to have their hands in disparate and diverse fields. The cohesion and unity of medicine, however, are found in its goals. Physicians employ methods and concepts of many disciplines in order to generate approaches and techniques that are peculiar to medicine. Medical science remains, as a result, a multiplicity-in-unity that is forever fluid and subject to modification and extension.[6]

Medicine as a Scientific and Humanistic Activity

Diverse and varied facets of human life contribute to health and illness, not merely those factors to which the natural sciences refer.[13] If medical practice is to promote health and ameliorate illness effectively, it must take all of these facets of life into account. We must reconceive medical science such that it can approach these manifold factors *scientifically*. And we so reconceive medical science when we view it as an employment of the critical attitude and the systematic search for evidence regarding these manifold factors.

Let us define "humanistic medicine" as that medical practice that focuses on the whole patient and not solely on the patient's disease.[4,6] Now we submit that such a humanistic medicine is identical with the scientific medical practice we have just delineated. A humanistic medicine must be a scientific medicine because both must take *all* the evidence bearing on the patient's health and illness into account. By contrast, a more narrowly based medical practice fails to be scientific as well as humanistic because it bypasses some of the directly given data, i.e., it ignores evidence regarding some of the factors that contribute to the patient's health and illness. Or if these other factors are taken into account in this more narrow practice, they are taken into account unscientifically, i.e., as "subjective factors" to be approached through "intuition" or "art."

How, then, does a scientific and humanistic doctor approach "the whole patient?" Scientific communicative interaction between the doctor and the patient insures that "the whole patient" is considered. In fact, when conceived scientifically and humanistically, the doctor-patient relationship is precisely communicative interaction. For communicative interaction creates a broad context within which manifold aspects of the patient's life are elicited, revealed, and tested through the acquisition of further evidence.[32,14,51] Only such communicative interaction can scientifically encompass all those components of the patient's life that bear on his or her health and illness; and therefore, only such interaction can prevent medical practice from shrinking into the narrow perspective of biomedicine.

Among those components of the patient's life that contribute to health and illness are the patient's own experience of illness,[15,52-56] the patient's hopes, fears, and expectations concerning the outcome of illness,[57,58] and the effect of illness on the patient's lived body.[49,50] The physician gains access to these so-called "subjective" factors through communicative understanding. But these factors are not "subjective" in the sense of being unscientific. The communicative understanding through which the doctor comes to appreciate the patient's experiences of illness can be fully scientific: this understanding can be firmly based on directly given data. In a fully scientific and humanistic medicine a central role must be found for detailed narratives of various illnesses as patients experience them.[59,60] There is also a need for pathographies, through accounts of the intertwining of illness with biography.[61] In addition, physicians should be carefully attuned to patients' hopes, fears, and expectations. These hopes, fears, and expectations have an impact on the course of illness and also on the willingness of patients to comply with bewildering or difficult treatment recommendations. And lastly, because of the pervasive influence of the spirit of abstraction, physicians may tend to think of the patient's body as merely the organism described by biology and neurophysiology. Yet however real and important the patient's organism may be for the medical practitioner, the patient's own prescientific experience of his or her body—what we have called "the lived body"—is also real and important. Through communicative understanding physicians must seek to grasp these various factors in their manifold interconnections.

Furthermore, communicative interaction between the doctor and the patient provides the broad context within which law-governed explanations can be situated. For, as we stressed earlier, explanations give us a special kind of technical power over some features of our patients' lives: such explanations allow us to subsume those features under general causal laws and thereby to predict and control outcomes. Not all those factors that contribute to health and illness can be approached in this manner, however. In fact, we only distort and misconceive these other factors if we attempt to force them into explanatory molds. Explanations thus apply to only various parts of "the whole patient." And for this reason explanations can play effective medical roles only within the larger context provided by communicative interaction.

In the manifold of evidence that must be elicited are, therefore, law-governed factors like laboratory test results and pathognomonic physical findings. It should be obvious by now that our quarrel with biomedical reductionism lies not in our denying the importance of this kind of evidence but rather with its exclusive focus on this limited sphere of evidence. And furthermore, we insist that the possibility for ordering the correct laboratory tests or observing the pathognomonic physical findings requires the broader context of communicative interaction. A. R. Luria, the great clinician and neuropsychologist, has similarly written,

I do not intend to underrate the role of instrumentation in medicine. But I am inclined to reject strongly an approach in which these auxiliary aids become the central method and in which their role as servant to clinical thought is reversed so that clinical reasoning follows instrumental data as a slave follows its master (p. 177).[10]

It may appear, however, that in some medical cases this comprehensive context of communicative interaction is not needed. After all, in certain situations, such as triage or mass screening, patients move, it seems, through a standardized processing in which they are treated like biological specimens or objects. And through this kind of processing certain diseases can be successfully diagnosed and treated. But even in these situations the broader context of communication and understanding remains fully operative: it is simply *presupposed* by both doctors and patients. It is *assumed*, for example, that patients, because of their expectations and understanding, are willing and able to cooperate and comply with such procedures and will thereby provide the necessary medical evidence. The fact that such willingness and ability is presupposed is demonstrated in cases in which patients prove to be unwilling or unable to comply. In those cases communication must first be established if the evidence is to be gathered.

Yet if communicative interaction restores breadth and largeness of scope to medical practice, how does it avoid becoming a conversation in which anything and everything in the patient's life becomes a relevant topic? Communicative interaction in medicine is circumscribed and delimited in four important ways:

1. In communicative interaction with the patient, the physician rigorously adopts a critical attitude, not the taken-for-granted attitude of everyday discussions. In such a process the patient says certain things that the physician must understand. Moreover, the patient behaves and gestures in certain ways that the doctor must interpret. The doctor also searches for physical findings and orders laboratory tests and procedures. These expressions, behaviors, gestures, findings, etc. are always examined within the critical attitude. Considered as an interconnected totality, they count as *evidence* of the patient's problem.

But like all scientific evidence, their meaning is not immediately obvious. Further evidence must be gathered in order to judge the meaning of previous evidence. And moreover, this evidence is considered in different ways. Certain features, such as expressions, behaviors, and gestures, are best evaluated through scientific understanding while other factors, such as laboratory test data, can be subjected to law-governed explanations.

As in every scientific endeavor, there must be ways to uncover or elicit the relevant evidence. Patients do not simply deliver this evidence in its totality and completeness. Because they too are human, patients may conceal some of this evidence or they themselves may not be aware of it. While patients may have certain expectations which must be taken into account, they will in all likelihood not even know what is relevant and what irrelevant. This means that the physician must have communicative skills for eliciting such evidence. And, on the other hand, physicians, because of components of their own personalities, may fail to examine patients adequately and may therefore bypass relevant evidence. In order to surmount this obstacle, physicians must learn to understand themselves better.

2. Communicative interaction in medicine always aims at and is delimited by the practical goals of promoting health and ameliorating illness. The doctor and patient take up solely those topics and examine solely those areas that may prove relevant to achieving these goals. Consequently, not just anything and everything will be discussed or investigated. Only aspects of the patient's life that relate to his or her health or illness will be considered. The medical interview, the physical examination, and laboratory tests and procedures are all guided and circumscribed by the practical goals of medicine.

3. The communicative interaction is always delineated and demarcated by the doctor's stock of peculiarly medical typifications, ideal types, and theories. These typifications, ideal types, and theories reduce the complexity of medical practice.[41] Without them, the broad approach we are endorsing would present an unmanageable complexity. Typifications, ideal types, and theories sharply circumscribe the possible options open to a physician when confronted with any patient. When, for exam-

ple, a knowledgeable neurologist or psychiatrist encounters a patient with a characteristic nervous, twitchy, eccentric, and noisy appearance, he or she may immediately typify the patient as a Touretter.[62] This typification leads to an examination of the patient in a particular direction. Furthermore, the physician's preconceptual typification is rapidly articulated as an ideal type: Tourette's syndrome. This ideal type explicitly identifies features for which the physician must search in the ensuing medical examination. As this examination moves further in this predelineated direction, evidence emerges that can confirm, disconfirm, or modify earlier conceptions.

Because of the physician's stock of typifications, theories, and ideal types, the skillful medical practitioner can always rely on a reasonably bounded repertoire of possible clinical approaches. Not just any and every approach will do. For example, an anxious, sweating patient who is breathlessly complaining of chest pain and clutching his chest is instantly typified as a person facing a cardiopulmonary emergency. Such typifications can immediately orient physicians and call forth characteristic protocols and procedures in the midst of urgent predicaments. In less dramatic circumstances, typifications and ideal types gleaned from chief complaints, salient physical findings, and tell-tale histories guide knowledgeable practitioners in directions appropriate for each case.

4. In clinical medicine, communicative interaction aims at appreciating patients *as unique, concrete individuals*.[35,40] Many of the conceptual, theoretical, and technical tools of medicine are general: they apply to all patients of a generic kind. But these tools, as they are actually used in clinical medicine, must be modified and particularized so that they come to apply to the patient as a concrete individual suffering from a specific problem. The generic typifications, ideal types, and theories of medicine function as the starting point of medical understanding; they are not the final point. Typifications, ideal types, and theories orient and guide clinical investigation *at the beginning*, but the ultimate goal for clinical investigators is an *individualized* understanding and treatment of the particular patient. Any law-governed explana-

tion of the patient's disease must be situated and utilized within the context of such individualized understanding. All of the manifold abstract perspectives used by the physician must converge on and render more precise the concrete problem facing the individual patient.

We may also formulate our position as follows. To the classical question, "Do physicians treat patients or diseases?" we would respond that physicians treat individual patients with diseases. The clinical genius of Oliver Sacks, for example, lies in his ability to appreciate the significance of such individualized understanding and treatment of patients. Medical approaches, concepts, and treatments, in Sacks' hands, are always adapted to the needs of particular patients.[62]

CONCLUSION

We have tried to sketch a comprehensive theory of medical practice which would be both scientific and humanistic. We call this theory "comprehensive" because we have sought to incorporate into it all the components of clinical medicine and we have attempted to show the relationships of these various components to one another. This includes even the dependence of medical practice on the prescientific lifeworld. This dependence is important because it highlights the concreteness of the patient's life that must be appreciated for both scientific and humanistic purposes. But at the same time we must see how the more abstract tools of medicine, such as law-governed explanations, can be situated within this concrete context and thereby perform their crucial functions. Forgetfulness of this broader context, however, uproots these abstract tools from their proper humanistic and scientific soil and leads to biomedical reductionism. Such a reductionism, we hope to have shown, is as unscientific as it is dehumanizing. Through a genuine appreciation of the biopsychosocial reality of the patient we can rehumanize our theory of medicine and still find an essential place for everything that biomedicine had correctly sought to stress.

REFERENCES

1. American Board of Internal Medicine. *A Guide to Awareness and Evaluation of Humanistic Qualities in the Internist.* Oregon, American Board of Internal Medicine, 1985.

2. Lipkin, M., Quill, T. E., Napodano, R. The Medical Interview: A Core Curriculum for Residencies in Internal Medicine. *Ann Int Med* 100:277–284, 1984.

3. AAMC Project Summary Report. Physicians for the Twenty-First Century. *J Med Educ* 59: 11, Part 2, 1984, p. 5.

4. Odegaard, C. *Dear Doctor: A Personal Letter to a Physician.* Menlo Park, Henry J. Kaiser Family Foundation, 1986.

5. Commentary on the GPEP Report. Commentary on the Report of the Panel on the General Professional Education of the Physician and College Preparation for Medicine. *J Med Educ* 61:345–352, 1986.

6. Schwartz, M. A. and Wiggins, O. P. Science, Humanism, and the Nature of Medical Practice: A Phenomenological View. *Perspect Biol Med* 28:331–361, 1985.

7. Engel, G. L. Physician-Scientists and Scientific Physicians: Resolving the Humanism-Science Dichotomy. *Am J Med* 82:107–111, 1987.

8. Engel, G. L. The Need for a New Medical Model: A Challenge for Biomedicine. *Science* 196:129–136, 1977.

9. Pellegrino, E. D. *Humanism and the Physician.* Knoxville, University of Tennessee Press, 1979.

10. Luria, A. R. *The Making of Mind: A Personal Account of Soviet Psychology.* Cambridge, Harvard University Press, 1979.

11. Eisenberg, L. Interfaces Between Medicine and Psychiatry. *Compre Psychiatry* 20:1–14, 1979.

12. Zaner, R. M. *The Context of Self: A Phenomenological Inquiry Using Medicine as a Clue.* Athens, Ohio University Press, 1981.

13. McHugh, P. R. and Slavney, P. R. *The Perspectives of Psychiatry*. Baltimore, Johns Hopkins University Press, 1983.

14. Cassell, E. J. *Talking with Patients 1: The Theory of Doctor-Patient Communication*. Cambridge, MIT Press, 1985.

15. Sacks, O. Clinical Tales. *Literature and Medicine* 5:14–19, 1986.

16. Gurwitsch, A. *Phenomenology and the Theory of Science*, edited by L. Embree. Evanston, Northwestern University Press, 1974.

17. Marcel, G. *Man Against Mass Society*. Translated by G. S. Fraser. Chicago, Regnery Press, 1962.

18. Whitehead, A. N. *Science and the Modern World*. New York, New American Library, 1948.

19. Husserl, E. *The Crisis of the European Sciences and Transcendental Phenomenology: An Introduction to Phenomenological Philosophy*. Translated by D. Carr. Evanston, Northwestern University Press, 1970.

20. Engel, G. L. The Clinical Application of the Biopsychosocial Model. *Am J Psychiatry* 137:535–544, 1980.

21. Baron, R. J. An Introduction to Medical Phenomenology: I Can't Hear You While I'm Listening. *Ann Int Med* 103:606–611, 1985.

22. Peterson, W. L., Sturdevant, R. A., Frankl, H. D. et al. Healing of Duodenal Ulcer with an Antacid Regimen. *New Engl J Med* 297:341–345, 1977.

23. Lauritsen, K., Rune, S. J., Bytzer, P. et. al. Effect of Omperazole and Cimetidine on Duodenal Ulcer: A Double Blind Comparative Trial. *New Engl J Med* 312:958–961, 1985.

24. Goldberg, M. A. Medical Treatment for Peptic Ulcer Disease: Is it Truly Efficacious? *Am J Med* 77:589–591, 1984.

25. Steer, M. L. and Silen, W. Diagnostic Procedures in Gastro-intestinal Hemorrhage. *New Engl J Med* 309:646–650, 1983.

26. Dronefield, M. W., McIllmurray, M. B., Ferguson, R., et al. A Prospective Randomized Trial of Endoscopy and Radiology in Acute Upper-Gastrointestinal Tract Bleeding. *Lancet* 1:1167–1169, 1977.

27. Peterson, W. L., Barnett, C. C., Smith, H. J. et al. Routine Early Endoscopy in Upper-Gastrointestinal Tract Bleeding: A Randomized Controlled Trial. *New Engl J Med* 304:925–929, 1981.

28. Merleau-Ponty, M. *Phenomenology of Perception.* Translated by C. Smith. New York, Humanities Press, 1962.

29. Weber, M. *Max Weber: Selections in Translation.* Edited by W. G. Runciman. Translated by E. Matthews. Cambridge, Cambridge University Press, 1978, pp. 7–32.

30. Jaspers, K. *General Psychopathology.* Translated by J. Hoenig and M. W. Hamilton. Chicago, University of Chicago Press, 1963.

31. Schutz, A. Common-Sense and Scientific Interpretation of Human Action. In M. Natanson (Ed), *Collected Papers I: The Problem of Social Reality* (pp 3–47). Martinus Nijhoff, The Hague, 1962.

32. Habermas, J. *The Theory of Communicative Action 1: Reason and the Rationalization of Society.* Translated by T. McCarthy. Boston, Beacon Press, 1981.

33. Husserl, E. *Experience and Judgment: Investigation in a Genealogy of Logic.* Translated by J. S. Churchill and K. Ameriks, Evanston, Northwestern University Press, 1973.

34. Schutz, A. Type and Eidos in Husserl's Late Philosophy. In I. Schutz (Ed), *Collected Papers III: Studies in Phenomenological Philosophy* (pp 92–115). The Hague, Martinus Nijhoff, 1966.

35. Schwartz, M. A. and Wiggins, O. P. Typifications: The

First Step for Clinical Diagnosis in Psychiatry. *J Nerv Ment Dis* 175:65–77, 1987.

36. Hanson, N. R. *Patterns of Discovery: An Inquiry into the Conceptual Foundations of Science.* Cambridge, Cambridge University Press, 1965.

37. Polanyi, M. *Personal Knowledge: Towards a Post-Critical Philosophy.* Chicago, University of Chicago Press, 1962.

38. Husserl, E. *Formal and Transcendental Logic.* Translated by D. Cairns. The Hague, Martinus Nijhoff, 1969.

39. Weber, M. *The Methodology of the Social Sciences.* New York, The Free Press, 1949.

40. Schwartz, M. A. and Wiggins, O. P. Diagnosis and Ideal Types: A Contribution to Psychiatric Classification. *Compr Psychiatry,* 28:277–291, 1987.

41. Schwartz, M. A. and Wiggins O. P. Systems and the Structuring of Meaning: Contributions to a Biopsychosocial Medicine. *Am J Psychiatry* 143:1213–1221, 1986.

42. Straus, E. *The Primary World of the Senses: A Vindication of Sensory Experience.* Translated by J. Needleman. London, Macmillan, 1963.

43. Ricoeur, P. *The Conflict of Interpretations: Essays in Hermeneutics.* Edited by D. Ihde. Evanston, Northwestern University Press, 1974.

44. Slavney, P. R. and McHugh, P. R. Life Stories and Meaningful Connections: Reflections on a Clinical Method in Psychiatry and Medicine. *Perspect Biol Med* 27:279–288, 1984.

45. Plessner, H. *Die Stüfen des Organischen und der Mensch, Gesammelte Schriften IV.* Frankfurt am Main, Suhrkamp Verlag, 1981.

46. Grene, M. Approaches to a Philosophical Biology. New York, Basic Books, 1968, pp. 55–118.

47. Hempel, C. G. *Aspects of Scientific Explanation and Other Es-*

says in the Philosophy of Science. New York, The Free Press, 1965.

48. Jonas, H. *The Phenomenon of Life: Towards a Philosophical Biology.* New York, Dell, 1966.

49. Leder, D. Medicine and Paradigms of Embodiment. *J Med Phil* 9:29–43, 1984.

50. Toombs, S. K. Illness and the Paradigm of Lived Body. *Theoretical Medicine* [in press].

51. Cassell, E. J. *Talking with Patients 2: Clinical Technique.* Cambridge, MIT Press, 1985.

52. Sacks, O. *Awakenings.* New York, Vintage Books, 1976.

53. Sacks, O. *A Leg to Stand On.* New York, Summit Books, 1984.

54. Stetten, D., Jr. Coping with Blindness. *New Engl J Med* 305:458–460, 1981.

55. Toombs, S. K. The Meaning of Illness: A Phenomenological Approach to the Physician-Patient Relationship. *J Med Phil* 12:219–240, 1987.

56. McWhinney, I. A. Are We on the Brink of a Major Transformation of Clinical Method? *CMAJ* 135:873–878, 1986.

57. Levenstein, J. H., McCraken, E. C., McWhinney, I. R. et al. The Patient-Centered Clinical Method. 1. A Model for the Doctor-Patient Interaction in Family Medicine. *Fam Pract* 3:24–30, 1986.

58. Brown, J., Stewart, M., McCraken, E. C. et al. The Patient-Centered Clinical Method. 2. Definition and Application *Fam Pract* 3:75–79, 1986.

59. Luria, A. R. *The Man With a Shattered World: The History of a Brain Wound.* Translated by L. Solotaroff, New York, Basic Books, 1972.

60. Jaspers, K. Jaspers on His Illness. In E. Ehrlich, L. H. Ehrlich, G. B. Pepper (Eds), *Karl Jaspers: Basic Philosophical*

Writings. (pp 528–534). Athens, Ohio, Ohio University Press, 1986.

61. Jaspers, K. *Strindberg and Van Gogh*. Translated by O. Grunow and D. Woloshin. Tucson, University of Arizona Press, 1977.

62. Sacks, O. *The Man Who Mistook His Wife for a Hat and Other Clinical Tales*. New York, Summit Books, 1985.

Reflections of a Post-Flexnerian Physician

by

G. Gayle Stephens, M.D.

You will have to forgive me for the presumptuousness of referring to myself as "post-Flexnerian." When I am finished you might want to classify me as "pre-Flexnerian," or worse, simply obsolete. However, I claim to have had a Flexnerian medical schooling—there was not any other kind when I attended, 1947–1952. I enjoyed medical school immensely and remember myself as a willing and basically uncritical student who was eager to do anything that my teachers assured me would make me a better doctor. As a freshman I read a novel about medical students at Johns Hopkins, *Miss Susie Slagle's*, that fired my romantic imagination about medicine in a way that has carried throughout my professional life. That book was the first I ever heard about Osler, Welch, Halstead, and Kelly. Medicine has been my mistress now for forty years, my source of personal identity, my window into the mysteries and secrets of human life, my benefactress in more ways than I can count. It's been a grand affair that still has power to charm.

Yet in many ways I am disenchanted, perhaps even apostate from Flexnerian medicine and its fierce, single-minded commitment to the most infinitesimal dimensions of human biology. The basic medical sciences, which Flexner loved and trusted so much, seem marginal to a great deal of what I find myself doing as a physician. I should acknowledge that I never really conquered the basic formulas of biological energy transformations. No shiny charts of metabolic pathways adorn my office walls; I display no icons to electron microscopy, DNA chemistry, immunogenetics, or cell membrane transport. I have never spliced a gene or created a monoclonal antibody. Receptors are as fantastic to me, and as much to be taken on faith, as electrons, quarks, and black holes. I would not recognize cyclic AMP if you showed me a gallon of it. I am shamefaced about these lacks and tremendously grateful to the discoverers of such knowledge, but in all honesty, I do not believe that learning the basic sciences over again in their modern form would add much to my functioning as a physician. Besides, I have had to learn a great many non-Flexnerian things in order to practice medicine. Therefore, I am no longer a completely faithful worshiper in the temple of Apollo; sometimes I bow at other altars and sacrifice to other gods.

Let me illustrate. The residents said that a recent lecturer in our department was fantastic. I had to hang on by my fingernails to keep from drowning in a torrent of data about the newest drugs for hypertension and heart failure. What they seemed to revel in, and asked good questions about, I had to clutch at, straining to recapture every fragment of memory about the pathophysiology and pharmacology of hypertension. Mutely, I sat at the end of the lecture, my head swirling with visions of molecules being cleaved and reassembled, enzymes activated and blocked, four kinds of adrenergic receptors agonized and antagonized, individually dissected renal tubules catheterized and perfused. Clearly, I was not comfortably "at home" in the geometric molecular world of renin, angiotensinogen I and II, prostaglandins and bradykinin, even though my medical career spans the entire history of modern anti-hypertensive pharmacotherapy.

I remember when no treatment was truly effective—barbiturates, bromides, nitrates, thiocyanates, and veatrum alkaloids—and recalcitrant hypertension was treated surgically by thoracolumbar sympathectomy. I remember the first excitement generated by hydralazine and ganglionic-blocking agents, powerful but dangerous, and the remarkable boon to office treatment when thiazides and Rawolfia alkaloids became available in the 1950s. Things are certainly better now, but I have seen therapeutic fads come and go, official recommendations revised repeatedly, educational campaigns for physicians and patients rise and decline, yet hypertension remains a major health problem and seems likely to continue.

There is a gap between what the molecular pharmacologists

know and the conquest of hypertension. Perhaps the obsolescence of my generation is part of the problem, but perhaps there is a human dimension to the treatment of hypertension that the pharmacologists overlooked or that their science is powerless against. Is there a sense in which the war against hypertension capsulizes both the strengths and weaknesses of Flexnerian medicine? It does not assuage my conscience to think so, but puts things into a better perspective. If pharmacology is necessary but not sufficient, there is surely some legitimacy in asking why and in thinking about what sufficiency requires.

Extra-Flexnerian Knowledge

Let us withhold concluding, for the moment, whether I am pre- or post-Flexnerian—I have surely disqualified myself as Flexnerian—yet I do claim to be a physician in good standing. My license has never been revoked and I see patients almost every day. I sincerely hope that I am not an imposter, a fraud, or a hopeless anachronism. Your judgment about that may depend upon whether I can go beyond my disenchantments and deficiencies and say in a more positive way what I know and do with and for patients. I hope that this will be more than an exercise in self-justification, since the issues being raised affect all physicians, especially those in direct patient care.

Since there is no orthodox Flexnerian science of the mind, much less of the self, the family, or the community, I have had to learn what I know about these from other sources. Patients, never merely bodies nor disembodied spirits, present themselves to physicians in exasperating wholeness, not realizing what dichotomous dilemmas they create for their physicians' science. They do not come in batallions, but one by one, always with connections to others, to society, and culture, which are also present by proxy and which cannot be ignored with impunity. A small proportion of patients are the bearers of well-defined Flexnerian diseases; most bear illnesses, the fear of disease, or simply questions about their health. I see very few who have no clinical concerns, no matter that they scheduled their appointments for "check-ups," whatever that turns out to mean.

I know that diseases, illnesses, and clinical problems occur within circumstances, contexts, and social systems that give meaning and to some extent definition to their forms. I have not only to do with pathological lesions that occur within the patient's skin, i.e., within tissue, but also within the self, and in the interstices of personhood. The late Michael Foucault correctly identified the beginning of scientific medicine with the concept of tissue,[1] and Flexnerian medicine has exploited that understanding brilliantly; but post-Flexnerian medicine must go beyond the geometry of tissue to psychic and social spaces where much of modern disease, illness and malaise reside.

Moreover, I know that illnesses of all sorts, not just mental disorders and behavioral problems, are not only matters of facts having logical and mathematical connections, as Flexner supposed and wrote, but they are also expressions of nonrational, irrational, and even absurd dimensions of human behavior. Simplistic notions of unitary causality will not suffice when the patient's actual historical existence must be taken into account. I get little explanatory power from the atomic theory, the cell theory, or the germ theory when what John Whitehorn called "man's pathogenicity for himself"[2] is the problem. Does anyone believe, for instance, that either the "causes" or the "effects" of AIDS have a Flexnerian solution, another magic bullet or vaccine, that will leave man's sexual behavior untouched?

KNOWING THE PATIENT

If there is one respect in which post-Flexnerian epistemology differs most from Flexnerian, it is in the relative importance of vision and hearing in knowing the patient clinically. Both, of course, are important and it seems a little silly to contrast them were it not for the fact that modern science seems preoccupied with visual imagery as the best and most valuable data. One chairman of a department of biochemistry was quoted recently as saying, "Life can be explained through biochemistry." Even with allowance for legitimate pride and homiletical extravagance, such an idea is fatuous. Walter J. Ong, Professor of English at St. Louis University, has pointed out that:

. . . the greatest shift in the way of conceiving knowledge between the ancient world and the modern world takes place in the movement from a pole where knowledge is conceived in terms of discourse and hearing and persons, to one where it is conceived in terms of observation and sight and objects. This shift dominates all others in Western intellectual history.[3]

To which Norris K. Smith, Professor of Art and Archeology at Washington University, St. Louis, replies that science through its preoccupation with observation, has come to worship the ideal of impersonal objectivity to the exclusion of other forms of knowing. He stated:

. . . let me suggest that in our day the most insidiously idolatrous kind of image-making ever known is also the commonest—to wit, photography. I find the notion ineradicably fixed in my students' minds that a well-focused camera reveals to us the truth about things—what my very worst students refer to as "reality as it really is" . . . The camera is widely thought to "see" with impartial accuracy, but in fact cannot see at all; for seeing is not a matter of optical mechanics; it is rather a process that involves our whole mental and spiritual being.[4]

The spoken word is the royal road to human understanding in medicine. It is the difference between "knowing that" or "knowing how" and "knowing whom" or "knowing whether." It is the difference between medicine as sophisticated veterinarianism and a distinctly human science and art. It is the difference between significance and meaning, observation and understanding; between a well functioning TV set and its program, a word processor and a novel.

I owe to Adolph Meyer the simple but profound idea that the physician must come to know the patient's name and the experience of life that the name stands for.[5] I owe to Samuel Novey the equally profound idea that the patient's history is invented as well as discovered.[6] L. J. Henderson (yes, he of Henderson-Hasselbach equation fame) taught me that the doctor and patient comprise a social system, a dyad, if you will;[7] and Harry Stack Sullivan was my source for understanding the structure and process of interviewing.[8] From George Herbert Mead and Talcott Parsons I have come to know the deeper dimensions of what Henderson meant by social system, the nature of the sick role, and the motivated character of symptoms.[9,10]

Michael Balint, to me the greatest in this list of teachers and the only one I ever met face to face, legitimized my life as a post-Flexnerian and gave me the courage and the tools to practice in that style.[11] Among many things he taught that patients turn their problems into illnesses, and that the physician's task is to turn illnesses back into problems. Martin Buber persuaded me that the highest form of human communication is the life of dialogue between subjects, not monologues between subjects and objects; that dialogue creates the possibility for genuine response to the other and sometimes "inflicts destiny upon us."[12] Leston Havens wrote that the first great task of medicine is to create a relationship with the patient and the second is to learn how to hear what that relationship reveals.[13] From Edmund Pellegrino I learned that the practice of medicine is foremost a moral enterprise in which "wounded humanity" seeks help from another.[14]

This "short list" of teachers and ideas by no means exhausts those to whom I owe homage. Let's consider it a symbol of a body of knowledge without which I could not possibly be a physician, one that could enrich any medical curriculum and move it beyond Flexnerian epistemology.

What I Do

Insofar as I am aware I see "run of the mill" patients who are not selected by their demographic characteristics, the nature of their clinical problems, or by my special interest or skills. Even if this is not literally true in all respects, I think of myself as a generalist who takes on all comers in the belief that I can offer them something, if not definitive care. My understanding of the generalist's role is precisely this; not that I must know or be able to do everything, but that I have a legitimate clinical interest in *anyone* who seeks my services. Not only that, but I also try to acknowledge whoever accompanies the patient to my office. I do not exclude from my rooms family members or friends who show an interest in the patient and to whom the patient appears to reciprocate. There is always time later when the patient can be seen alone. These "others" often turn out to be important sources of information or play crucial roles in the outcome of the visit.

Without intending to exaggerate, romanticize, or sentimentalize my work with patients, it must be obvious by now that my chief sources of knowledge about patients are the spoken word and the doctor-patient relationship. I try with everyone to form a therapeutic alliance, though I do not always succeed. Failure in this provides painful but important opportunities for learning.

So I begin and end every consultation with a patient with conversation that in its best moments becomes dialogue. I come to know patients, bit by bit, only as we disclose ourselves to each other in a trusting relationship. This is the reverse of the way we come to know the natural world; we gather facts and then we trust their orderliness and come to say that we know an object. In truth we know *about* the object, we know *that*. Such knowing will not do in human relationships, whether of friends, lovers, or parents and children. Here we have to trust first and later come to know whom.

These ideas lend an aura of mystery and expectancy to the meeting of patient and physician. Rarely do I fail to feel it. There is a golden, almost sacred, moment at the beginning of each interview when anything is possible if I do not, by my biases, preoccupations, or impatience, distort or misguide it. A "tone" will be set in the first few minutes that determines what I am likely to come to know.

Conversation and dialogue do not allow me to escape the fact that in some respects the relationship between physician and patient is ambiguous, ambivalent, and even adversarial. I do not agree with Thomas Szasz that the physician's traditionally-assumed benevolence towards the patient is actually fraudulent and that self-interest or interest in objective truth always takes precedence over interest in the patient's welfare. Neither do I agree that the physician's proper role is that of expert, whose primary duty is to tell the truth, letting the chips fall where they may. I acknowledge, however, that the patient's interests and the physician's are sometimes obscure, lack congruence, and may even be conflicted, especially now that so many physicians are employed by others than the patient. This is an important moral problem that needs constant attention, but is not necessarily the most important way in which physicians and patients fail to understand each other or have common goals.

A REAL RELATIONSHIP

The spoken word is notoriously subtle and testimony is not the same as evidence. Pauline Bart has noted unique ethnic and cultural qualities of "vocabularies of complaint."[15] If patients couch their complaints in concrete terms, physicians are apt to respond in concrete ways. Balint and others have taught me that complaints are often "tickets of admission" to the physician's office, and Feinstein emphasized the importance of the "iatrotrophic stimulus" as the reason for the visit that may lie behind the stated complaint.[16] Moreover, the meaning and purpose of the complaint may not be entirely clear to the patient. Balint wrote about the time when the patient is alone with the illness before consulting a physician, the time when the illness is being organized or is in gestation. Parsons described the motivated nature of complaints, that they serve a more or less well-defined purpose. Sometimes I think that physicians have overemphasized the unconscious or metaphorical character of complaints and failed to explore fully their conscious elements. A great deal of attention has been paid in recent years to the quality of the physician's communications to the patient, especially as this has become formalized in the legal doctrine of informed consent. Our ancestors also emphasized the need for clarity and full disclosure on the part of the patient and this idea was contained in the earliest Code of Ethics of the AMA in a section titled "The Patient's Duties To The Physician." This section has been omitted in recent versions of the Code.

John Berger, in his penetrating study of the British general practitioner John Sassall, described the transformation that occurs in the professional lives of many physicians from "life saver" to "healer," wherein the key is the physician's capacity and willingness to use his or her own imagination to encounter the patient's.[17] This is a non-Flexnerian skill in that its subject matter is not the law-abiding regularities of nature, but the caprices of culture as assimilated by the individual. W. R. Houston quoted below on the placebo effect, also noted that the physician does not necessarily believe what the patient believes about the illness.[18]

The physician–patient relationship is at least as complex and ambivalent as any other intimate human relationship. It takes time and energy and delicacy to cultivate. Like marriage, it is not a state to be entered lightly or unadvisedly. So I always begin by believing the patient and taking the complaints at face value, even if, later, I have to confront the incongruities. I am not a surveyor, a poll-taker, an interrogator, or a prosecuting attorney; I do not merely collect data towards which I am affectively neutral or a dispassionate observer. Often I must disclose myself in the process of coming to understand a patient. There is no way to keep the meeting completely safe for me if it is not equally safe for the patient. Both must take the risks of getting to know the other when medicine is practiced in the most effective way.

THERAPEUTICS

I have a small repertoire of technical and procedural skills and I use a small pharmacopeia of drugs. I have no confidence in a purely objective therapeutics that "works" regardless of who applies it or in what context it is applied. W. R. Houston wrote, in the 1930s, that the placebo has always been the norm of medical practice, and while I do not self-consciously use drugs as placebos I certainly try to maximize the placebo effect of myself. He also wrote, "The faith that heals, heals not through argument but by contagion." Michael Balint also wrote lucidly about the doctor as a "drug." Such notions may well be pre-Flexnerian, but they have not been obviated by scientific medicine.

I consider myself a familiar (in the sense of an intimate, confidential, associate or spirit) of the human body, especially in its macro dimensions. I have day to day close contact with it; look at, touch, and smell it, probing its intimate spaces, directly sensing its various effluvia. I know its beauty and grotesqueness, its asymmetries, leanness, and fatness, its lumps and bumps, all its orifices. More than that, I know its anatomy uncommonly well.

I can tell when it is functioning well and when and in what ways it is impaired. My fingers can usually locate its pain and tenderness and I rarely fail to palpate the part that hurts. I can ordinarily guess what lies beneath its surface, although sometimes I have to resort to endoscopy and the marvels of modern imaging. It might be too much to say that I love the body, but I have great respect for it and for the person's it is. My style of medical practice would be impossible without direct access to the living body. I make a point of this only because I sense a trend in modern medicine to distancing from the body, to know it mainly indirectly by means of instruments, machines, or chemical analyses, and to assign unpleasant or routine contact with the body to others. I would not welcome a future technology that obviated the physical examination.

For the most part I do not hurt my patients. I try not to inflict pain during my examinations and procedures. I'd like to think of my medicine as gentle and nonviolent. I warn patients when something I am about to do might hurt and give them permission to say, "Stop!" Most of all I try to reduce the risks of causing iatrogenic illnesses. I prescribe drugs cautiously and in as small doses as possible, warning of possible reactions, and avoiding known interactions. I am careful about recommending invasive diagnostic procedures, which are so easily available nowadays. The average physician is only a telephone call away from a vast array of tests and procedures that formerly required referral to a sub-specialist. Now the subspecialists are likely to refer patients to the same radiologists that are available to me. I can order a myelogram, four-vessel cerebral angiography, or a CAT scan with contrast as easily as a neurosurgeon. Pathologists will do a bone marrow examination for me as well as for a hematologist. The power to invade the patient's body is limited only by the physician's conscience and judgment. The ancient adage, "First, do no harm" has never been more important.

On the other hand, I am eager to relieve symptoms, pain and suffering. My risks are on the side of relieving inappropriately, of overusing analgesics, tranquilizers, antidepressants, and the like. I worry a lot about creating drug dependency and I spend a lot of time talking with patients about drugs and their proper use. Sometimes I have to be confrontive about prescription refills.

I allow a certain amount of dependency upon me. I am not very good at setting strict limits on my time and energy. I am vulnerable to being "conned," to give the demanding or exploitive patient the benefit of the doubt. I tend to take the patient's side in matters of conflict with insurance companies, employers, "the government" or other bureaucracies. I give permission to be sick, to miss work, to stay home from school, to be excused from gym class. I feel little compunction to protect the system from the patient. Short of direct lying, cheating or stealing I am apt to support a patient's claim for disability, or to word a diagnosis so that the insurance company will pay for a claim.

I do not feel compelled to demand perfection in my patients, to challenge every habit, every compromise, every adaptation to illness. I do not require that they always choose the best. I try to give sound counsel, but I do not break relationships when patients choose not to take it. I respect their right to say, "No," to give up, even to die. This does not mean that I have no interest in what my patients choose, but I will try to help them through whatever they choose.

My errors are likely to be those of omission rather than commission, of doing too little rather than too much. I hold on, I wait, I "buy" time. I know that "mother nature" is on the side of most healers and that many illnesses improve with time. I do not see myself mainly as a "disease fighter" or a "death defier." I do not believe that death is the worst enemy. I feel very bad if I miss a diagnosis of cancer, fail to prevent a heart attack or stroke, or overlook a rare disease, but I am not willing to organize my entire practice around avoiding these mistakes.

Sometimes I violate a patient's confidentiality, particularly when the problem involves intimate others. I value openness, seek permission, and try to persuade patients to share their secrets with family members and others who care, have responsibility, could be affected adversely by the illness, or who may be in complicity with the illness. I do not refuse to take a telephone call from a worried spouse or an anxious parent. If I believe that illness and healing both occur within personal and social contexts, I cannot accept confidentiality as an absolute value. On the other hand, I am not above using confidentiality to protect patients from institutions and organizations. If this sounds paternal, so be it; I am willing to be bound to the same sort of judgment when I am the patient.

Sometimes I become overinvolved with patients and my own subjectivity becomes a problem. Whether one calls this identification, counter-transference, ignorance, immaturity, or lack of common sense, it is the price of doing business. I do not ever expect to get over it, though I do not enjoy the pain of a neurotic or broken relationship, professional or otherwise. I have simply given up the Flexnerian ideal of complete objectivity, which was always an idolatrous delusion wrapped in layers of denial, hiding the distance between physicians and patients.

WHAT'S THE POINT?

Why labor these points? Not to recreate the mystery and magic of a more superstitious era; not to return to the dogmatism, empiricism, and sectarianism that Flexner so thoroughly despised; not to repudiate the scientific knowledge that has been so arduously and expensively amassed during the past 75 years. Not at all! The reason is to insure that the power of medicine does not become demonic, that medicine retains its roots as a servant rather than a master of individual and public goods. It is only within the small contexts of millions of physician-patient relationships that are open, safe, and mutually determined that the public has any chance of controlling and protecting itself from its own Promethean propensities. If war is too important to be left to generals, health is surely too important to be left to an impersonal professionalism that is bound to become coercive as it becomes more authoritarian. If the twentieth century has learned anything about Science, it surely is that Science is not socially, politically, or morally neutral. The biological sciences, no less than physics and engineering, must be kept under "civilian" control. Such control is an issue in every physician-patient encounter. The pure science of medical knowledge must be tempered by other forms of human knowing, and for its own good, should always be subject to judgment within a larger frame of reference than itself.

Educational Implications

In reciting these claims and confessions about how I practice medicine and what sorts of knowledge I take to be important, I expose myself to criticism from both Flexnerians and those who want to reform that system. To the former I am hopeless anti-scientific; to the latter I lack the courage to be radical enough. However, my personal characteristics are not the real issue; I am merely one example of a type of professional development that must engage all experienced physicians if they are to fill in the vacuums of their formal medical education. If I am idiosyncratic in my adaptations and compromises, if we all are more or less idiosyncratic in our understanding of the deeper dimensions of the physician's work, it is because our formal systems of medical education have either left this part to chance, deliberately ig-nored it, or actually opposed it. I tend to believe all three. We would not have participated in the dialogue at Wickenburg if there were not powerful and stubborn forces at work in medical education that keep it focused on producing what a dean of my acquaintance likes to call "superb human biologists," and what I prefer to call human veterinarianism. (No disrespect for veteri-nary science or animals intended.)

Our medical schools are not weak and ineffectual. Flexnerian reforms created a remarkably effective system of education that is almost impossible to resist. It is elite, lock-step and over-whelming; if it fails in one or more respects, it is not by accident, but by choice. The benefits of Flexnerian medicine are unargua-ble, but it has flaws that must be acknowledged and redressed. It is time that the nation's medical schools accept responsibility for *all* their effects, the good and the bad. It has always been amazing to me how medical school faculties can disassociate themselves from the characteristics of doctors and organized medicine that they profess to deplore. There are no physicians who were not first students, few who were not residents for three or more years. There is a direct and continuous connection between what medical schools believe, teach, and approve and the characteristics of medical practice and the behavior of organized medicine. The schools must take the bitter with the sweet and realize that these are two sides of the same coin.

Flexnerian medicine is alive and well in 1987, fueled by the energy of the surgical specialties, transplant technology, immunogenetics, and spectacular advances in body imaging. There is no sign that a "Kuhnian paradigm shift" is anywhere in sight in the basic medical sciences, even though that has been a wishful thought in some quarters for twenty years or more. The "body as a machine" metaphor seems still to have a great deal of explanatory power, and medical research, in the main, is still committed to it. Yet in the wake of medicine's conspicuous successes there are genuine problems with its science that promise to become even more significant in the decades just ahead, problems for which no technological fix seems possible. Medicine's best successes have come in those conditions for which the germ theory, the atomic theory, and the cell theory are most applicable. Alfred North Whitehead once observed that all Western philosophy can be considered footnotes to Plato.[19] Similarly, the major medical advances in the twentieth century are footnotes to Lister, Virchow, and Pasteur. No other classes of disease than the infectious diseases and their analogs may truly be said to have been "conquered," and even this task is incomplete, as the AIDS epidemic exposes so dramatically. Moreover, new illnesses that do not fit neatly into the pathologists' taxonomies have emerged as major unsolved problems—violence of all sorts, mental disorders, addictions, stress, sexual problems, abortions, care of the aged, etc. etc.—problems that John Whitehorn said originate in man's pathogenicity for himself. What a litany of unfinished business!

Some might say that such problems are not truly medical, or not only medical, but medicine, in one way or another has staked a claim on them. It may be correct that we have medicalized too much, bitten off more than we can chew, but even that propensity can be attributed to the *hubris* of Flexnerian medicine and its confident optimism that every illness can be made to fit its theories and methods. Perhaps hubris, what theologians call overwhelming pride, is the most egregious flaw in modern medicine. It is the flaw that blinds us to flaws, hides us from the real nature of medical fallibility, and obscures our understanding of the limits of science. It keeps us from seeking and receiving help from sources outside medicine.

One of the ironies of the Flexnerian reforms is the ambiguous relationships between medical schools and universities. On one hand universities became the new proprietors as private, for-profit schools disappeared; but the dream of integrated basic science faculties and interdisciplinary learning was never realized. In many instances medical schools developed in urban settings at some distance from their parent universities, and all of them showed a remarkable propensity for becoming the tail that wags the dog. Their independent development was abetted by the power and popularity of medical science plus their ability to generate funds, first from public and private sources, more recently from payment for medical practice. There is a lamentable chasm between the faculties of medical schools and other schools in their universities, which accounts, in part, for the intellectual one-sidedness and academic isolation of medicine from other relevant disciplines.

Oddly enough, it is the basic science departments in medical schools that are the most isolated from the academic social sciences and the humanities, and whose faculties are the most resistant to curricular changes that might repair the deficiencies of Flexnerian medicine. They fight tenaciously for their piece of the curricular pie, object to the early introduction of clinical information, and oppose elective courses or volunteer learning experiences on the grounds that *any* infringement on the students' free time is a threat to their immersion in the basic medical sciences. Small wonder that physicians have become more expert and less learned than Flexner would have liked. The first two years in medical school are not unlike a horse race in which the students, like thoroughbreds wearing blinders, run as fast as they can towards a finish line that includes passing an examination (NBME Part I) having a built-in failure rate of 11–13 percent. One wonders, in view of declining applications to medical schools and the skyrocketing costs of tuition, how long it will take medical students to realize that they now have the power to demand something different and better. There can be little doubt that Flexnerian medical education for 75 years has been run by a feudalistic bureaucracy.

What all this means to me is that no superficial changes in the education of physicians are likely to produce broadly literate physicians who are better prepared to deal with the clinical problems that are already apparent and that will be even more important in the twenty-first century. It also means that Flexnerian medicine, like dogmatic medicine and empiricism before it, is not likely to be able to heal itself.

Unfortunately, current changes in medical practice will not contribute to the necessary reforms. The industrialization and privatization of medicine are no reforms at all, but the mere extension of a narrowly conceived Scientism into the organization and management of medical practice. We have no reason to hope that corporation morality will be any better in medicine than it is in defense contracting or on Wall Street. A medical-industrial complex can be no more self-regulatory and socially responsive than the military-industrial complex that President Eisenhower warned us about so presciently.

From where I sit, the philosophical beliefs and attitudes of medical educators, the problems of clinical practice, and the organization and structures of medical care have common root defects that were contained in Flexner's famous report.[20] They are the preoccupation with the human body as the only proper object of medical knowledge and the faith in experimental biology as the solution to all problems of health and illness. Until we take the whole human person in his or her social and cultural dimensions as the proper object of knowledge, until we expand our notions of science to include forms of rationality other than the logical, we will continue to depersonalize and fragment medical care, increase its costs beyond all calculation, and fail to make all its benefits equally available to the whole population. I do not expect that Flexnerian medicine will come to a grinding halt; perhaps a minority of physicians and other professionals should have a primary commitment to it, but it should not be allowed to exclude all other forms of knowing and it should not dominate the entire medical profession and the schools that produce the professionals.

Flexner likened the thinking of a physician to that of an engineer, but with more urgent decisiveness for the life and death of individuals. I prefer to believe that a physician also needs the creativity and intuitiveness of the novelist, but be that as it may, the relations between physics and engineering might be a good model for future development of the medical sciences. We need theoretical physicists, and I would not mind if they comprised an elite in status and pay, but I would not want them designing all our roads and bridges or overseeing the manufacture of all our industrial products. Similarly, we need human biologists who are committed to the canons of positivist science, but the applied medical sciences cannot be based entirely on that. Physics had to confront its moral limitations in the Manhattan Project and it has never been the same since. Scientific medicine is headed for the same impasse. Let us hope it sees itself clearly before we are all ushered into a "brave new world" that none of us really wants.

REFERENCES

1. Foucault, M. *The Birth of The Clinic: An Archeology of Medical Perception* (translated from the French by A. M. Sheridan Smith). New York, Vintage Books, 1974.

2. Whitehorn, J. "The Doctor's Image of Man." New Engl J Med 265:301, 1961

3. Ong, W. (Quoted in No. 4).

4. Smith, N. "The Idolatry of Objectivity." *Washington University Magazine* 51:4, Winter 1981, pp 13–17.

5. Meyer, A., *Collected Papers of Adolph Meyer.* E. Winters, Ed. Baltimore, Johns Hopkins Press, 1951.

6. Novey, S. *The Second Look: The Reconstruction of Personal History in Psychiatry and Psychoanalysis.* Baltimore, Johns Hopkins Press, 1968.

7. Henderson, L. *L. J. Henderson on The Social System.* B. Bar-

ber, Ed. Chicago and London, The University of Chicago Press, 1970.

8. Sullivan, H. *The Psychiatric Interview.* New York, W. W. Norton & Co. Inc., 1954.

9. Mead, G. Strauss, A. Ed. *George Herbert Mead on Social Psychology.* Chicago and London, The University of Chicago Press, 1956.

10. Parsons, T. *Social Structure and Personality.* London, The Free Press, Collier-Macmillan, LTD, 1964.

11. Balint, M. *The Doctor, His Patient, and the Illness.* New York, International Universities Press Inc., 1957.

12. Buber, M. *Between Man and Man.* New York, The Macmillan Company, 1965.

13. Havens, L. The Anatomy of a Suicide. *New Engl J Med* 272:401, 1965.

14. Pellegrino, E. *The Philosophical Basis of Medical Practice.* Oxford University Press, 1981.

15. Bart, P. Social Structure and Vocabularies of Discomfort: Whatever Happened to Female Hysteria? *J Health and Social Behavior* 9:88, Sept. 1968.

16. Feinstein, A. *Clinical Judgment.* Baltimore, Williams & Wilkins, 1967.

17. Berger, J. and Mohr, J. *A Fortunate Man: The Story of a Country Doctor.* London, Writers and Readers Publishing Cooperative, 1976.

18. Houston, W. The Doctor Himself as a Therapeutic Agent. *Ann Int Med* 11:1416, 1938.

19. Whitehead, A. *Process and Reality.* New York, Harper & Brothers, 1960.

20. Flexner, A. *The Flexner Report on Medical Education in the United States and Canada,* 1910. Reprinted by Science & Health Publications, 1960.

Science in Medicine:
Too Much or Too Little and Too Limited in Scope?

by

Leon Eisenberg, M.D.

It has become commonplace to hear it said, not only by the laity, but by medical students and physicians as well, that there is too much science in medical education. Indeed, some teachers of basic science believe such a view underlies *Physicians for the 21st Century*, the Report of the Panel on the General Professional Education of the Physician and College Preparation for Medicine. That interpretation was specifically rejected in the commentary on the Report adopted by the Executive Council of the Association of American Medical Colleges,[1] but many academics remain uneasy. The public seems to yearn for the icon of the physician portrayed in Sir Luke Fildes' "The Doctor," a physician, let us remember, who could do little more than be a comforting presence at the bedside while his young patient's illness ran its course.

Still, are those of us who celebrate the contribution of science to medicine merely deluding ourselves that the recent history of clinical medicine is one of progress? Is it the case that the doctor of yesteryear was kinder and more compassionate than his successors have proved to be? Why, in John Knowles' trenchant phrase,[2] are we "doing better and feeling worse"?

The Application of Science to the Clinic

Paul Beeson[3] undertook the instructive task of comparing the treatments recommended in the first (1927) edition of *Cecil's Textbook of Medicine* with those in its 14th (1975) edition, by which time Beeson and McDermott had become its editors. By contemporary standards, Beeson rated the value of 60 percent of the remedies in the first edition as harmful, dubious or merely symptomatic; only 3 percent provided fully effective treatment or prevention. In the 48-year interval between the two editions, effective regimens had increased sevenfold and the dubious ones had decreased by two-thirds. The evidence led him to the conclusion:

> Substantial advances have been made along the whole frontier of medical treatment. The patient today is likely to be treated more effectively, to be returned to normal activity more quickly, and to have a better chance of survival than 50 years ago (p. 84).

The motor behind these accomplishments has been the systematic application of the basic biomedical sciences to the investigation of disease. Although research in the natural sciences began to exert a shaping influence on medical theory in the last half of the nineteenth century, it did not have a major impact on medical practice until the 1940s. It was not until then that laboratory findings had been translated into diagnostic and therapeutic methods. Today, we have entered an era in which the rate of advance in fundamental science is rapidly accelerating; the time lag between discovery and application has been remarkably shortened. Consider only what has become possible through the use of recombinant DNA methods employing restriction fragment length polymorphisms (RFLPs).[4] I cite them to highlight the continuing fruitfulness of "reductionistic science"—when that reductionism is applied to appropriately chosen problems. Just this February (1987), two sets of papers reported important new research on the biological substrate of (a) manic depressive disorder and (b) Alzheimer's disease.

Egeland and coworkers[5] demonstrated, in an Old Amish kindred, linkage between the major locus for bipolar disease and the loci for insulin and the oncogene Ha-*ras*-1 on chromosome 11. It is presumably not coincidental that the marker genes on chromosome 11 are also closely linked to the gene encoding tyrosine hydroxylase, the principal enzyme in the synthesis of catecholamine neurotransmitters. In the same issue of *Nature*, two other research groups found no evidence for such a linkage in 3 Icelandic[6] and 3 non-Amish American[7] kindreds characterized by autosomal dominant transmission of bipolar disease. What these reports establish is the heterogeneity of the inherited diathesis for affective disorders; there must be at least two different sets of genes that confer risk. Furthermore, the genetic evidence from the Old Amish pedigree, rather than precluding a role for environmental precipitants of manic depressive disease, provides new possibilities for their specification. The ability to detect persons at risk through RFLPs in informative family kindreds permits the design of studies to identify the environmental factors which result in expression (penetrance) only in some and phenocopies in still others.

In the same month, *Science* published reports of equally exciting contributions to an understanding of the biology of Alzheimer's disease. St. George-Hyslop and coworkers[8] obtained data tracing the defective gene to chromosome 21 in autosomal dominant familial Alzheimer's disease (FAD). Two other research groups[9,10] demonstrated that the gene coding for beta amyloid protein, which accumulates in the brains of Alzheimer's patients and of older Down's patients, also maps to chromosome 21. Provocative as these findings are, the FAD gene may not be identical with the gene coding for beta amyloid protein; moreover, the FAD gene proved *not* to be on the region of chromosome 21 which, when present in a third copy, leads to Down's syndrome. Three weeks after these reports, Delabar et al.,[11] using a cDNA probe to determine the dosage of the beta amyloid protein gene on chromosome 21 in patients with sporadic Alzheimer's disease, with trisomy 21 Down's and karyotypically normal Down's, found evidence for gene duplication in leukocyte DNA from all three sets of patients. Whether the duplication is either necessary or sufficient to account for Alzheimer's disease is yet to be determined. For all the ambiguity in the interpretation of these findings, they represent a considerable advance in the understanding of Alzheimer's disease, whose incidence is increasing as more Americans survive to the age of risk and whose prevalence grows even faster as we become more expert at postponing death.[12] Any hope of preventing Alzheimer's disease or controlling its course rests on fundamental research in neurobiology.

The very success of biomedicine has exacted a price in the way it has narrowed the physician's focus exclusively to the biology

of disease. However, the remedy does not lie in abandoning reductionism where it is appropriate but in incorporating it within
a larger social framework to enable the physician to attend to the
patient as well as to the disease. As an intellectual bridge over the
chasm between molecular biology and social science, let us turn
now to the uses of clinical epidemiology in identifying and analyzing contemporary therapeutic dilemmas.

RESEARCH ON MEDICAL PRACTICE

The problem is apparent in everyday medical practice, during
which physicians make decisions to recommend standard treatments whose effectiveness they take for granted. The extent of
variation in physician judgment was not recognized until the
methods of clinical epidemiology were applied to study the rates
at which procedures were being employed. The findings identified marked variability which was not attributable to differences
in morbidity in the populations surveyed. In the absence of a
sound data base, physicians follow local "custom" because they
are unaware of the uncertainties besetting their judgments.

Wennberg and his colleagues[13] documented the extent of variation in rates for surgical procedures among small geographic
areas with comparable populations. In a survey of the New England states, rates for tonsillectomy were found to vary sevenfold and those for hysterectomy and prostatectomy four-fold
from one area to another. In research on the Medicare population, similar patterns of variation in the performance of surgery
have been demonstrated; for example, rates for coronary artery
bypass surgery range from a low of 7 to a high of 23 per 10,000
from one region of the U.S. to another.[14]

There is a remarkable parallel between the number of surgeons per population and the rates for operative procedures
across countries: both figures are about twice as high for the
U.S. as for the U.K., with Canada about halfway between the
two.[15] However, these data do *not* tell us whether the U.S. is
oversupplied, the U.K. undersupplied, or Canada about right.

The problem is not simply the pecuniary interest of physicians
working in a fee-for-service system. In a comparison among

Norway, the U.K., and the New England states, surgical rates showed similar variability *within* each country despite the differences in rates *between* countries and in the methods of organizing and financing medical care among them.[16] These findings contrast with relatively small variations in rates for appendectomy, regarded as the only acceptable treatment for a presumptive diagnosis of appendicitis. That there are differences between surgeons is evident, not only from geographic variations, but also from second opinion studies which have found that about one-quarter of patients for whom surgery is recommended by one surgeon have that opinion reversed by a second.[17] If U.K. rates for the seven common operations examined by Wennberg and his colleagues had applied to the U.S., deaths associated with surgery would have decreased by a third to a half.[18]

Unnecessary and unduly prolonged hospitalization in itself results in serious health risks. More than 3 million infections are acquired each year in U.S. hospitals, afflicting almost one patient in every 18 admitted to an acute care facility.[19] In one study of 815 consecutive patients on a general medical service of a university hospital,[20] 36 percent experienced an iatrogenic illness, most instances arising from drugs or invasive procedures. In 9 percent of all patients admitted, a major untoward incident occurred; in 2 percent, it was thought to have been a factor contributing to the patient's death!

What options are there to change this unsatisfactory state of affairs? By having specialty colleges specify the indications for particular procedures[21] and by feeding back information to local practitioners on area variations,[22] it has been demonstrated that surgical rates can be reduced. Yet such steps do no more than reify expert opinion. Professional consensus can be no better than the quality of the evidence on which it is based; for many medical and surgical procedures the available data are equivocal. As Vayda and Mindell point out,[23] "the issue of necessary versus unnecessary surgery will not be resolved until the question of efficacy or effectiveness of competing treatments (or treatment versus nontreatment) is answered." For that we will need: systematic collation of available information; randomized clinical trials to evaluate treatments of uncertain efficacy; and a mechanism to change physician behavior to accord with the best available evidence.

Technology or Science?

Some critics conclude from the apparent over-reliance on technical procedures that medical practice suffers from "too much science." That criticism confuses science with technology and mistakes biomedical science for the only science relevant for medicine. Lewis Thomas[24] has stressed that:

> . . . These technologies are, in their very existence, the best of arguments for more basic biological research . . . Unless we learn the . . . causes of coronary occlusion, and . . . how to prevent it, the artificial heart will be in production . . . costing the moon and impossible to prohibit.

The misuse of technology stems from such factors as: a medical payment system that pays doctors more the more they perform procedures; the legal and moral controversies that make it difficult for doctors to withdraw "lifesaving measures," which do no more than prolong the process of dying; and the failure of medical education to prepare doctors to weigh competing claims.

The current reimbursement scales of the fee-for-service system reward procedures with fees far higher than those for time spent in clinical assessment. A gastroenterologist realizes a net hourly income from endoscopy that is more than six times greater than from the general management of the patient's illness.[25] The disproportion between the fees paid for procedures and those for a thorough history and physical examination is transforming gastroenterologists into endoscopists[26] and cardiologists into "catheterologists."[27] The fact that the net income of technically oriented specialists is much higher than that of primary care practitioners influences the career choices of young physicians and contributes to the disproportion in the ratio between generalists and specialists. A change in the relative fee schedule is necessary to provide an economic incentive to expand primary care, including a greater emphasis on disease prevention and health promotion.

Therapeutic advances accentuate moral dilemmas. Whereas once doctors could do nothing for a patient with pneumococcal pneumonia but await the outcome of the disease process, we now possess powerful antibiotics that make a decisive difference. This is an extraordinary accomplishment when the life saved is a life of quality. But is it for the good when medicine intercepts the terminal illness that might have brought a merciful end to pain and misery? The ability of cardiorespiratory assist to maintain vegetative existence in such patients has confronted society with unprecedented ethical dilemmas. Now that death can be postponed, it has been transformed from an event of nature to a human decision. Yet, does it make sense to indict the technology that can restore meaningful life because it can also be employed to make death an agonizing process? The issues at stake are not technical, but moral and legal; the resolution of the dilemma requires input from doctors, but ultimately rests with society at large.

The third factor leading to the misuse of technology is the inability of many practitioners to weigh competing claims. All too many medical graduates have not mastered the rudiments of biostatistics and decision theory. Without reasonable proficiency in the logic of scientific inference and the methods of statistics, practitioners lack the tools to assess the conclusions drawn in medical articles. How else are we to understand the persistence of carotid endarterectomies or the rush to embrace radial keratotomies in the absence of evidence to justify their use? Doctors have an altogether unwarranted faith in the reliability of clinical methods and tests.[28] How else are we to explain the indifference to matters of sensitivity and specificity in ordering tests and evaluating test findings[29] without weighing *a priori* probabilities? The fact is that medical education, far from being "too scientific," suffers from too much emphasis on memorizing evanescent "facts" and too little on science as a way of framing questions and gathering evidence.

THE ROLE OF THE SOCIAL SCIENCES

The ultimate measure of the effectiveness of medical care is its impact on the health status of the population it serves. Existing patterns of medical practice do not provide information on the denominator; that is, the relevant population from whom the sample seen in the office is drawn. The fact is that community surveys regularly identify many more symptomatic persons and many more with abnormal physical findings than are under medical care.[30,31] By having individuals in the community complete a daily health diary, Demers et al.[32] found that only a small minority of self-identified illness episodes resulted in going to the doctor; the vast majority were managed within the family or by the use of "alternative" practitioners. In the presence of life stress, symptoms are not only more likely to be experienced but also more often lead to medical consultations.[33,34] Unfamiliar with these fundamental findings, physicians are ill prepared to identify the sources of patient distress and instead focus their attention (and that of their patients) on inappropriate diagnostic and therapeutic measures. Moreover, failure to recognize depressive syndromes manifested by means of somatic symptoms is all too common in medical practice;[35] it reflects serious inadequacies in the preparation of physicians for primary care practice.[36]

The education doctors receive is so narrowly focused on individual case management that they have lost sight of their responsibility to the community they serve. Even in Britain, where all citizens are assured coverage by a national health service, general practitioners limit their responsibility to the patients who consult them and overlook those in their panel who are silent,[37] thus missing the opportunity to promote and monitor the health of the population. Medical education must be broadened to include the concepts and methods of social epidemiology.

The pattern of disease characteristic of a particular society is a function of its level of development. Consider the changes in disease epidemiology in the United States. In 1900, the three leading causes of death were infectious: pneumonia, tuberculosis and diarrheal disease. By 1940, they had declined sharply and had been displaced by increasing rates of heart disease, cancer and cerebrovascular disease.[38] The decline in mortality from infectious disease resulted from improvements in sanitary engineering, housing, hygiene and nutrition during an era when there had been few advances in medical therapeutics; the new pattern of mortality arose from changes in diet, physical activity, smoking and exposure to environmental toxins, as well as from the graying of the population, as more people live into the age of risk for chronic diseases.

These statistics only begin the analysis of health needs within the population. The distressing fact is that morbidity and mortality are inversely correlated with social class; persons with the lowest income and the least education have the greatest need but are allocated fewer resources for their health care even in a country with a National Health Service, such as the United Kingdom.[39] A Task Force of the U.S. Department of Health and Human Services identified a gap of 5.6 years in life expectancy between whites and blacks and a black mortality rate more than 40 percent higher than that for whites.[40] The six most important contributors to the disparity were heart disease and stroke, homicides and accidents, cancer and infant mortality, which can be reduced by public health preventive measures and timely medical care.

Confronted by lives lost in such epidemic proportions, we would do well to recall the words of Rudolf Virchow, written almost a century and a half ago:

> If disease is an expression of individual life under unfavorable conditions, then epidemics must be indicative of mass disturbances of mass life.

The resolution of such "mass disturbances of mass life" demands measures well beyond those of medicine as such. Nevertheless, medicine, which Virchow identified as a social science, has a major role to play in identifying their consequences, studying their sources, and advocating the social remedies.[41]

Just as sociology can help physicians to recognize the role of class and social organization as disease determinants at the macro level, social anthropology enables the physician to understand that illness, patienthood, and health-related behaviors are social constructions that biology does not account for. I have elsewhere proposed the usefulness of distinguishing between "disease" and "illness," terms used synonymously in ordinary usage.[42] Physicians have been taught to conceptualize diseases as abnormalities in the structure and function of body organs and tissues. But patients suffer illnesses; that is, experiences of disvalued changes in states of being and in social function. Disease and illness do not stand in a one-to-one relationship. Similar degrees of organ pathology can generate quite different reports of pain and distress; illness may occur in the absence of detectable disease; the course of the disease is distinct from the trajectory of the accompanying illness. A visit to the doctor may be more likely, on average, when disease is present; although being diseased, feeling ill and being a patient may overlap, they are not coterminous.[43]

Furthermore, life circumstances have a profound effect on disease risk through their influence on host resistance. When the counties of North Carolina were ranked on an index of social disorganization, the stroke mortality rate (disaggregated by age) for black men proved to be highest in the tier of counties in the highest quintile on social disruption.[40] Similar results were obtained for rates of hypertension among blacks in a survey of Detroit census tracts.[45] Ruberman et al.[46] studied cumulative mortality following myocardial infarction among patients enrolled in a trial of beta-blockers; mortality proved to be highest among those with the least education, the most life stress and the greatest social isolation.

Nuckolls et al.[47] tracked a cohort of white married primiparae of similar age and social class with measurements of life change scores (a proxy for stress) and social support. Life change and social support each had an independent effect on the risk for the complications of pregnancy, with high life change increasing, and high support decreasing, the risk; in effect, social support buffered the pregnant woman against stress. Brown and Harris[48] studied the social ecology of psychiatric disorder among women in London. Rates for depression proved to be severalfold higher among working class than middle class women. Moreover, among those in the working class, depression was found more often among those with three or more children under age 14 in the home, with no outside employment, and without an intimate or confiding relationship with a husband or boyfriend; that is, one in which feelings were shared, whether or not sexual intimacy also occurred. In all groups, rates were higher when the individual had experienced threatening life events in the 9 months before the onset of illness.

The way a given culture conceptualizes illness and the behaviors it prescribes for curing or preventing it must be taken into account if even the best of what medicine has to offer is to be effective. This is most readily evident in efforts to apply Western biomedicine in the Third World. Chen and his colleagues[49,50] have reported the disappointing results they obtained after applying an effective and appropriate technology, tetanus vaccine, to the prevention of infant deaths in Bangladesh. Two years after its introduction, the vaccine, a simple measure which can be delivered to pregnant women in their homes with a biologic efficacy of 100 percent, had reduced net infant mortality by less than 3 percent; yet, epidemiologic studies had demonstrated that neonatal tetanus accounts for 26 percent of all infant deaths. Less than a quarter of the pregnant women had accepted the vaccine because local experience had not persuaded the villagers of its effectiveness. Bangladeshi folk terms for diseases that afflict infants do not distinguish neonatal tetanus from other fatal conditions. Because deaths from these other causes continued despite vaccine administration, its "perceived efficacy" was far less than its actual efficacy against tetanus.

Postneonatal mortality is higher among female than among male children in Bangladesh, a reversal of the sex ratio found in the West. The explanation for this phenomenon lies in the preference extended to sons in the allocation of the limited resources available to the family. In apportioning family meals, mothers give smaller rations to their daughters than to their sons (who contribute more to family earnings even as children and who will be the economic support for their parents in old age). Where undernutrition is endemic, this additional restriction on food intake leads to greater malnutrition in girls and to lower resistance to infection. Further, parents more often take a sick son than a sick daughter to the clinic, even when it is free, because of resource costs; i.e., hours of work lost during travel.[51]

These examples make clear the vital importance of understanding the complex interactions between technology and culture, if the methods of biomedicine, so successful in a Western context, are to meet the health needs of the Third World. As Lincoln Chen[52] has pointed out:

> Future research should attempt to incorporate the strengths of the natural and social sciences. The biomedical sciences focus on medical causes of disease and death, often disregarding the sociopolitical, environmental, and behavioral forces that powerfully shape disease risk and therapeutic response. The social sciences, in contrast, usually correlate mortality with socioeconomic indicators without an understanding of how such forces generate disease risk and the biological processes leading to disease outcome. Policies based on only [one] or the other type of discipline tend to be either too technology based (biomedical) or broad (and often vague) in approach.

I could go on to list the importance of: economic analysis for an understanding of resource allocation; history for an essential perspective on the development of medical theory and practice; social psychology for the illumination of the doctor-patient relationship, and so on. These matters have been reviewed elsewhere.[53]

What Were the Virtues of the Old-Fashioned Family Doctor?

Let me return to the question I raised at the outset: is it true that the "old-fashioned family doctor" was more responsive to patient needs than his successors have proved to be? Mind you, I do not contend that doctors today—or yesterday, for that matter—are—or were—as aware of the personal and social issues in patient care as they should be; to the contrary, it is my thesis that a key function of systematic instruction in the social sciences is to address that failing. But were things better once upon a time? If not, whence stems the belief that they were?

The fact is that complaints about practitioners being "too scientific" date from well before applied science had any appreciable impact on medical practice. Professor Francis W. Peabody wrote in 1923:[54]

> The layman of the older generation . . . who feels that something has been lacking in the way of warmth, sympathy and understanding . . . is very

apt to hark back to earlier days. "What we need," he says, "is a general practitioner!"[1](p. 7)

. . . Older practitioners complain that young graduates . . . are too scientific and do not know how to take care of patients. (p. 27)

Why the call for the general practitioner of earlier days? What had changed? Peabody provides the clue:

The more a doctor knows of his patient's general background, the greater advantage he has in handling the case . . .[The general practitioner] knows the patient from childhood up—his physical health, the nervous and mental strain to which he has been subjected, the conditions of his social, business and domestic life, and more even than this, he may have the same detailed knowledge of the patient's parents and of the circumstances of their lives . . . (p. 30)

The virtues of the family doctor Peabody spoke to stemmed from an intimate acquaintance with patient, family and community over years of practice, and *not* from formal instruction received in medical school. Those virtues were inherent in the doctor's role in an America of small towns, family farms and multigenerational families, an America that was disappearing as he wrote. Generalist or specialist, today's physician no longer has the chance to know the extended family over several generations, with one in five American families moving every year; familiarity with "the conditions of the patient's social, business and domestic life" is no longer automatically accessible to "neighborhood" doctors now that our population has shifted to a predominantly urban locus, with its anonymity and fragmentation.

The task for contemporary medical education is to teach physicians to obtain, through systematic and sensitive inquiry, that knowledge of the patient's "social, business and domestic life" that astute practitioners once acquired through long acquaintance with family and community. The problem isn't with what doctors are taught but what they aren't taught and never were:

1. Indeed, a century before Peabody, we find in Balzac's novel *Pere Goriot*, written in 1834, a passage that might have been written today: Bianchon, reassuring his friend Rastignac that he cares for the dying Goriot, comments: "Doctors already in practice see only the illness; I can still see the sick man, my boy."

to understand the intimate interconnections between health and illness, on the one hand, and the way men and women live in society and what they believe, on the other. Preparation for medical practice in an increasingly pluralistic society requires knowledge of and respect for cultural differences. More than that, it demands the acquisition of skills in assessing needs and negotiating common understandings with individuals and families. Patients differ in their values, their beliefs about health and illness and their expectations of the doctor's role.[55]

It is not enough to mean well. The doctor must know enough to *do* well for the patient. That requires as deep an understanding of the social sciences as of the biological sciences.

THE BARRIERS TO IMPLEMENTATION

What are the barriers to a more widespread incorporation of humanistic and psychologically responsive care into medical practice? Without denying that some physicians do care for patients in this way, why is it that so many do not? The barriers, I suggest, stem from the following elements: acquired insensitivity; skepticism about the "reality" of psychosocial factors; misattribution of therapeutic effects; difficulty in learning new skills; and the current social context of medical practice.

ACQUIRED INSENSITIVITY

Certain aspects of proper medical care all agree to be desirable arise from claims that are irrelevant to effectiveness in a narrow medical sense. Treating patients with respect, giving them scheduled appointments, providing amenities in the clinic, keeping the clinic open evenings for patients who work, and allowing time to listen and reflect are right and proper on grounds of simple decency, whether or not it has been demonstrated that they lead to disease control. Failure to disprove the "null hypothesis" in a randomized trial would not alter their propriety. They stand on their own as dicta to guide human relationships without requiring pragmatic justification.

Why is responsiveness to these issues not universal? The reasons are not far to seek. Responsiveness costs money. It reduces "efficiency." It demands that the doctor value the patient's time equally with his or her own. The dignity of patients is given short shrift in the public institutions where doctors are trained. The bureaucratic structure of hospitals and clinics is organized to facilitate internal operations and to preserve staff privileges. When doctors define their task as the correction of biologic derangements, it should be no cause for surprise that the psychosocial aspects of patient care are put on the back burner. Students model themselves on what they see. Bianchon, the student, can still see "the sick man"; Bianchon, the doctor, will have learned to see "only the illness"—in order to get his job done expeditiously. The flaw is not in the students we recruit; it is in what they learn from us.

Indeed, a case can be made for the proposition that the formal content of the curriculum (much of which is forgotten by the time of graduation) has less impact on the kind of physicians students will become than the covert curriculum; that is, the values the curriculum implicitly embodies (by what is *not* taught as well as by what is), the behaviors modeled by the faculty, and the rewards and admonishments given to students. Taken together, they constitute a powerful social press for conformity with extant professional values, given the eagerness with which students have sought admission and the prestige and income they foresee once they pass the hurdles. Socialization may be what education is all about. A century later, American medical schools continue to follow the 1893 Hopkins model of four years of college, an exacting admissions process, and four years of medical school[2] despite change in the nominal content of courses. Research by social scientists offers a penetrating analysis of professional socialization;[57-61] the findings appear to have had little influence on medical education, perhaps because social science, a critical discipline by its very nature, is practiced by "outsiders"

2. Indeed, the recognition that four years has magic properties for the production of reliable physicians dates back at least as far as the medieval English universities, if not to the first great medical school, founded in Salerno in the eleventh century.[56]

with no clout in the power structure of medicine. Yet, it is only social science research that can help us to move beyond asserting personal bias in debates on medical education.

SKEPTICISM ABOUT THE "REALITY" OF PSYCHOSOCIAL FACTORS

Efficacy is a proper major concern of practicing physicians. Many psychosocial interventions are advocated on the grounds that they will lead to better outcomes. One such is the proposition that a sensitively ascertained history and a carefully done physical examination will often lead to the correct diagnosis without dependence on an extensive battery of costly, often superfluous and sometimes risky tests.[62] Early recognition and appropriate management of psychosocial problems yield better outcomes with fewer visits and less hazard than the endless search for a biological will-o'-the-wisp in patients who somatize distress.[63] Why, then, does such evidence not persuade more physicians to modify their practice styles?

There is widespread skepticism among physicians as to whether psychological and social factors are as "real" as biological ones.[64] Classroom exercises will have convinced all of them of the power of biological reductionism. It is not only that so much more time is devoted to the natural as opposed to the "unnatural" sciences in medical education, but that the elegance of molecular biology is so much greater. Contrast the detail in which it is now possible to describe the pathophysiology of the thalassemias—from errors in the genome, through variant hemoglobin structures, to clinical manifestations[65]—with what can be said about the pathophysiologic link between social isolation and mortality risk.

Berkman and Syme[66] have demonstrated that patients in the lowest quartile on a social network index experienced more than two times the mortality of those in the highest quartile during a nine year interval. That is a solid fact and a very important one for medical practice, because it has relevance for all patients and not merely those with a relatively uncommon genetic disease. However, the mechanisms by which social isolation translates into disease risk remains a matter for surmise. To be sure, that doesn't alter the power of the phenomenon one whit. But because being able to describe the pathophysiology of disease is so central to the culture of biomedicine, physicians continue to be skeptics about social research, when they are not downright arrogant in their dismissal of it.[67]

MISATTRIBUTION OF THERAPEUTIC EFFECTS

Most patients treated by most doctors get better most of the time. In part, this stems from the self-limited nature of most illness episodes, in part from the positive expectancies aroused by the medical encounter.[68] However, because transactions between doctors and patients are mediated by procedures and medications, doctors attribute the benefits obtained to the remedies prescribed and fail to recognize the role of ritual and symbolism in healing. This unacknowledged bonus for medical practice is treated as "experimental noise" in pharmacologic research. Placebos are employed in clinical trials as proxies for expectancy effects in order to parse out the "specific" actions of drugs. Because the drug is the focus of inquiry, equally specific patient and doctor effects are left unaccounted for.

Consider the findings of a randomized double blind clinical trial of clofibrate.[69] Among the men in the "active drug" arm of the study, those who took their pills regularly had a significantly lower five year mortality than did non-compliers (15.0 percent versus 24.6 percent). However, among the men receiving a lactose placebo, those who took their pills experienced an equally large reduction in mortality as compared to poor compliers (15.1 percent versus 28.3 percent). Because the focus of the study was on the drug, the investigators concluded that: "these findings . . . show the serious difficulty . . . of evaluating efficacy in subgroups determined by patient responses . . ." (p. 1038)[69]. How bizarre to downplay the demonstration of a highly significant mortality effect associated with compliance, an effect so large it would have caused the stock of a pharmaceutical company to soar, had the difference been attributable to the medication! It was precisely the restricted focus of the research to the collection of data on traditional medical variables that made it impossible to account for the outcome in terms of traits which may have been associated with compliance (such as social class, cigarette smoking, alcohol consumption, diet, exercise or other health habits or beliefs).

Under certain circumstances, *not* receiving a placebo can influence outcome. In a study my colleagues and I carried out some years ago at a training school for delinquents,[70] we administered either a psychotropic drug or a matched placebo to the youngsters in an experimental cottage. As a reference point in assessing stability in behavior ratings by house parents, we administered no treatment in a cottage we naively designated as a "control." Behavior improved steadily among the experimental subjects, whether they were on drug or placebo; in contrast, ratings in the "control" cottage progressively worsened and culminated in a mass elopement. After the fact, we discovered that the youngsters as well as their caretakers in this second residence were angry at not receiving a treatment that they believed would shorten the time to return home. Our designation of those individuals as "controls" did not correspond with their self-definition as persons cheated of perceived benefit.

Until the psychosocial context of the encounter between doctor and patient is given explicit attention in research and teaching, doctors will be as mystified as their patients about the ingredients of effective medical care.

UNLEARNING OLD HABITS

Psychosocial interventions do not lead to dramatic changes in outcome that are immediately evident to the individual physician; they are discernible only over time and with a large enough patient sample. For example, as many as 10 percent of patients counseled by physicians to stop smoking do in fact stop.[71] It is possible to read the findings as "no more than" 10 percent and dismiss counseling as ineffective by the standard expected of most interventions. On the other hand, once we recall that some 60 million Americans still smoke, 10 percent amounts to some 6 million persons who might be spared the hazards associated with cigarettes if all doctors, rather than just a minority, took their public health responsibility seriously. When a disease is life threatening and a treatment effect dramatic, physicians are ready to adopt the new treatment at once, particularly when it requires no more of them than prescribing one drug rather than another. When changing from one treatment method to another involves unlearning old habits and acquiring new skills, change is painful and slow in coming.

Franz Kafka[72] has epitomized the problem in a sentence from his short story, *The Country Doctor*:

> To write prescriptions is easy but to come to an understanding with people is hard.

Doctors are trained to "do something." They believe[73] that patients expect a consultation to have a tangible outcome: a pill or a shot. It requires the disruption of overlearned habits to change from doing to listening (and to come to recognize that listening is an important way of doing). It demands a shift in paradigms from disease to illness in order to change from prescribing to attending to meanings and to helping patients to examine options. Despite the fact that it is primary care physicians to whom patients with psychosocial disorders turn and from whom they get such help as they receive,[74] most practitioners report themselves ill-trained for the task, uncomfortable with it, and reluctant to undertake it. Educated in tertiary care centers, they are poorly prepared for the problems patients present in primary care.

The Social Context of Medical Practice

Robert Ebert (p. 97),[75] in commenting on the Western Reserve experiment in medical education, had this to say about the limits to curriculum reform:

> Nonmedical school forces are far more important in shaping the character and career plans of young physicians than anything that happens to them during the four years of medical school.

However much skepticism and lack of training may contribute to the problem, the most decisive determinant of physician failure to incorporate a psychosocial approach into practice stems from the perversity of current reimbursement schemes.

As noted, physicians are rewarded disproportionately when they perform procedures in contrast to providing "cognitive services." One need not suppose that physicians are solely motivated by economics to recognize that it is difficult to resist the temptation to carry out a procedure, if only to confirm a clinical diagnosis, when it yields greater income and at the same time impresses the patient with its magical properties. What is essential is implementation of a reimbursement scheme that is technology-neutral, a scheme that leaves the decision to employ procedures to clinical judgement rather than to the pocketbook. Even the family physician, with little technology to command, soon discovers that taking the time to listen to patients and to explore their lives with them reduces income sharply. This long standing problem has been exacerbated by Medicare and Medicaid fee schedules which can only be described as mean, both in motive and in effect for patient and physician.[76]

The current emphasis in national health policy on controlling costs rather than on enhancing health outcomes inexorably ratchets down on the provision of comprehensive care. It can only promote cynicism among our students if we preach humanism and ignore the realities of the contemporary scene[77]: admissions policies designed to unload the "losers" onto county hospitals; house officers overwhelmed by more admissions and sicker patients; "sicker and quicker" discharges dictated by fixation on the bottom line; the deliberate "demarketing" of unprofitable services: the squeeze on outpatient clinics to increase throughput (i.e., income); and resistance to quality control rationalized in the rhetoric of clinical freedom.

Let me be explicit about our responsibility as faculty members.

Do we mean what we say when we urge students to attend to the personhood of the patient? Then, when we conduct teaching rounds, we must visit the bedside and ask the patient how he feels and what his illness means to him; we undercut our words when we limit our questions to house officers about lab values and differential diagnosis in conference rooms off the wards.

Do we want our house officers to care for their patients? Then, let us begin by caring for interns and residents; it is intolerable that we exploit them as cheap labor, reprimand them for error, but rarely praise them for accomplishment.

Is informed consent a ritual formula designed to meet the legal requirements of the record or is it a process through which we validate the autonomy of the patient? If the latter, then we must take the time to demonstrate to our students how the information the patient needs to have can be presented clearly and, often, more than once, in order that the doctor can support the patient's right to choose among alternatives.

Do we really believe in improving standards of care? Then, we must support quality controls with teeth to them and be prepared to have our own practices subjected to close scrutiny.

Do we really mean what we say about the importance of equity and access for all in health care? Then, we must become visible to our students as social activists in behalf of the 37 million Americans without health care coverage. What is unconscionable is silence on the matter when the academic medical centers we serve rationalize retreat from justice in language and concepts borrowed from the marketplace.[78]

Unless we put as much energy into the effort to change the social context in which our graduates will practice as we do into curriculum reform, we will have betrayed the very principles we profess. Our patients and our students deserve better of us.

REFERENCES

1. AAMC Executive Council: Commentary on the Report of the Panel on the General Professional Education of the Physician and College Preparation for Medicine. *J Med Educ* 61:346–352, 1986.

2. Knowles, J. (ed.) *Doing Better and Feeling Worse: Health in the United States.* New York, W. W. Norton and Co., Inc., 1977.

3. Beeson, P. B. Changes in medical therapy during the past half century. *Medicine* 59:79–99, 1980.

4. Kan, Y. W. and Dozy, A. M. Polymorphism of the human beta-globin structural gene: relationship to sickle mutation. *Proc Natl Acad Sci USA* 75:5631–5635, 1978.

5. Egeland, J. A., Gerhard, D. S., Pauls, D. L. et al. Bipolar affective disorders linked to DNA markers on chromosome 11. *Nature* 325:783–787, 1987.

6. Hodgkinson, S., Sherrington, R., Gurling, H. et al. Molecular genetic evidence for heterogeneity in manic depression. *Nature* 325:805–806, 1987.

7. Detera-Wadleigh, S. D., Berrettini, W. H., Goldin, L. R. et al. Close linkage of c-Harvey-*ras*-1 and the insulin gene to affective disorder is ruled out in three North American pedigrees. *Nature* 325:806–808, 1987.

8. St. George-Hyslop, P. H., Tanzi, R. E., Polinsky, R. J. et al. The genetic defect causing familial Alzheimer's disease maps on chromosome 21. *Science* 235:885–890, 1987.

9. Goldgaber, D., Lerman, M. I., McBride, O. W. et al. Characterization and chromosomal localization of a cDNA encoding amyloid of Alzheimer's disease. *Science* 235:877–880, 1987.

10. Tanzi, R. E., Gusella, J. F., Watkins, P. C. et al. Amyloid beta-protein gene: cDNA, mRNA distribution, and genetic linkage near the Alzheimer locus. *Science* 235:880–884, 1987.

11. Delabar, J. M., Goldgaber, D., Lamour, Y. et al. Beta amyloid gene duplication in Alzheimer's disease and karyotypically normal Down's syndrome. *Science* 235:1390–1392, 1987.

12. Gruenberg, E. M. The failures of success. *Milbank Mem Fund Quart* 55:3–24, 1977.

13. Wennberg, J. E. and Gittelson, A. Variations in medical care among small areas. *Scient Amer* 126:120–134, 1982.

14. Chassin, M. R., Brook, R. H., Park, R. E. et al. Variations in the use of medical and surgical services by the Medicare population. *New Eng J Med* 315:285–290, 1986.

15. Vayda, E., Mindell, W. R. and Rutkow, I. M. A decade of

surgery in Canada, England and Wales and the United States. *Arch. Surg.* 117:846–853, 1982.

16. McPherson, K., Wennberg, J., Hovind, O. et al. Small area variations in the use of common surgical procedures: an international comparison of New England, England and Norway. *New Eng J Med* 307:1310–1314, 1982.

17. McCarthy, E. G. and Finkel, M. L. Second opinion elective surgery programs: outcome status over time. *Med Care* 16:984–994, 1978.

18. Wennberg, J. E., Bunker, J. P. and Barnes, B. A. The need for assessing outcomes of common medical practices. *Ann Rev Pub Health* 1:277–295, 1980.

19. Haley, R. W., Culver, D. H., White, J. W. et al. The nationwide nosocomial infection rate: a new need for vital statistics. *Am J Epidem* 121:159–167, 1985.

20. Steel, K., Gertman, P. M., Crescenzi, C. et al. Iatrogenic illness on a general medical service at a university hospital. *New Eng J Med* 304:638–642, 1981.

21. Dyck, F. J., Murphy, F. A., Murphy, J. K. et al. Effect of surveillance on the number of hysterectomies in the Province of Saskatchewan. *New Eng J Med* 296:1326–1328, 1977.

22. Wennberg, J. E., Blowers, L., Parker, R. et al. Changes in tonsillectomy rates associated with feedback and review. *Pediat* 59:821–826, 1977.

23. Vayda, E. and Mindell, W. R. Variations in operative rates. *Surg Clin NA* 62:627–639, 1982.

24. Thomas, L. Whitehead Institute Inaugural Address. 5 December 1984.

25. Almy, T. P. The role of the primary physician and the health care "industry." *New Eng J Med* 304:225–228, 1981.

26. Spiro, H. M. My kingdom for a camera—some comments

on medical technology. *New Eng J Med* 291:1070–1072, 1974.

27. Phibbs, B., The abuse of coronary arteriography. *New Eng J Med* 301:1394–1396, 1979.

28. Koran, L. M. Reliability of clinical methods, data and judgements. *New Eng J Med* 293:642–650; 696–701, 1975.

29. Casscells, W., Schoenberger, A. and Grayboys, T. B. Interpretation by physicians of clinical laboratory results. *New Eng J Med* 299:999–1001, 1978.

30. White, K. L., Williams, T. F. and Greenberg, B. G. The ecology of medical care. *New Eng J Med* 265:885–892, 1961.

31. Mechanic, D. and Newton, M. Some problems in the analysis of morbidity data. *J Chronic Dis* 18:569–580, 1965.

32. Demers, R., Altamore, R., Mustin, H. et al. An exploration of the depths and dimensions of illness behavior. *J Fam Pract* 11:1085–1092, 1980.

33. Tessler, R., Mechanic, D. and Dimond, M. The effect of psychological disease on physician utilization: a prospective study. *J Health Soc Behav* 17:353–364, 1976.

34. Mechanic, D. Effects of psychological distress on perceptions of physical health and utilization of medical and psychiatric facilities. *J Human Stress* 4:26–32, 1978.

35. Katon, W., Kleinman, A. and Rosen, G. Depression and somatization. *Amer J Med* 72:127–135; 241–247, 1982.

36. Kleinman, A. The cultural meanings and social uses of illness. *J Fam Pract* 16:539–545, 1983.

37. Hart, J. T. A New type of general practitioner. *Lancet* ii:27–29, 1983.

38. Levy, R. I. and Moskowitz, J. Cardiovascular research: decades of progress, a decade of promise. *Science* 217:121–129, 1985.

39. Department of Health and Social Security. *Inequalities in Health: Report of a Research Working Group*. London, 1980.

40. The Secretary's Task Force. *Report on Black and Minority Health*. Washington, D.C., U.S. Department of Health and Human Services, August 1985.

41. Eisenberg, L. Rudolf Ludwig Karl Virchow, where are you now that we need you? *Amer J Med* 77:524–532, 1984.

42. Eisenberg, L. Disease and illness: distinctions between professional and popular ideas of sickness. *Culture, Medicine and Psychiatry* 1:9–23, 1977.

43. Eisenberg, L. What makes persons "patients" and patients "well"? *Amer J Med* 69:277–286, 1980.

44. Neser, W. B., Tyroler, H. A. and Cassel, J. C. Social disorganization and stroke mortality in the Black population of North Carolina. *Amer J Epidemiol* 93:166–175, 1971.

45. Harburg, E., Erfurt, J. C., Chape, C. et al. Socio-ecologic stressor areas and Black-White blood pressure: Detroit. *J Chronic Dis* 26:595–611, 1973.

46. Ruberman, W., Weinblatt, E., Goldberg, J. et al. Psychosocial influences on mortality after myocardial infarction. *New Eng J Med* 311:552–559, 1984.

47. Nuckolls, K. B., Cassel, J., Kaplan, B. H. Psychosocial assets, life crisis and the prognosis of pregnancy. *Amer J Epidemiol* 95:431–441, 1972.

48. Brown, G. W. and Harris, T. *Social Origins of Depression: A Study of Psychiatric Disorder in Women*. New York, Free Press, 1978.

49. Rahman, M., Chen, L. C., Chakraborty, J. et al. Tetanus toxoid: I: Reduction of neonatal mortality by immunization of non-pregnant women and women during pregnancy in rural Bangladesh. *Bull WHO* 60:261–267, 1982.

50. Rahman, M., Chen, L. C., Chkraborty, J. et al. Tetanus

toxoid II: Factors related to immunization acceptance among pregnant women in a maternal-child health program in rural Bangladesh. *Bull WHO* 60:269–277, 1982.

51. Chen, L. C., Huq, E., and D'Souza, S. Sex bias in the family allocation of food and health care in rural Bangladesh. *Pop Dev Rev* 7:54–70, 1981.

52. Chen, L. C. Primary health care in developing countries: overcoming operational, technical, and social barriers. *Lancet* ii:1260–1265, 1986.

53. Eisenberg, L. and Kleinman, A. *The Relevance of Social Science for Medicine*. Boston, D. Reidel Publishing Co., 1981.

54. Peabody, F. W. *Doctor and Patient*. New York, Macmillan Company, 1930.

55. Harwood, A. (ed.). *Ethnicity and Medical Care*. Cambridge, Harvard University Press, 1981.

56. Talbot, C. H. *Medicine in Medieval England*. New York, American Elsevier Publishing Co., 1967, Chapter V, pp. 64–71.

57. Becker, H. and Geer, B. The fate of idealism in medical school. *Am Sociol Rev* 23:50–56, 1958.

58.. Bosk, C. *Forgive and Remember*. Chicago, University of Chicago Press, 1979.

59. Mumford, E. *Interns: From Students to Physicians*. Cambridge, Harvard University Press, 1970.

60. Freidson, E. *Professional Dominance*. New York, Atherton Press, 1970.

61. Freidson, E. *Doctoring Together: A Study of Professional Social Control*. Chicago, University of Chicago Press, 1975.

62. Hampton, J. R., Harrison, M. J. G., Mitchell, J. R. A. et al. Relative contributions of history-taking, physical examination, and laboratory investigation to diagnosis and manage-

ment of medical outpatients. *Brit Med J* i:486–489, 1975 (May 31).

63. Mumford, E., Schlesinger, H. J., Glass, G. V. et al. A new look at evidence about reduced cost medical utilization following mental health treatment. *Amer J Psychiat* 141:1145–1158, 1984.

64. Eisenberg, L. Mindlessness and brainlessness in psychiatry. *Brit J Psych* 148:497–508, 1986.

65. Weatherall, D. J. and Clegg, J. B. *The Thalassemia Syndromes.* Oxford, Blackwell Scientific Publications, 1981.

66. Berkman, L. F. and Symes, S. L. Social networks, host resistance and mortality: a nine year follow-up study of Alameda County residents. *Am J Epidemiol* 109:186–204, 1979.

67. Petersdorf, R. G. and Feinstein, A. R. An informal appraisal of the current status of "medical sociology." See Ref. 53, pp. 27–48.

68. Frank, J. D. *Persuasion and Healing* (revised edition). New York, Schocken Books, 1974.

69. Coronary Drug Project Group. Influence of adherence to treatment and response of cholesterol on mortality in the Coronary Drug Project. *New Eng J Med* 303:1038–1041, 1980.

70. Molling, P. A., Lockner, A. W., Sauls, R. J. et al. Committed delinquent boys: the impact of perphenazine and placebo. *Arch Gen Psychiat* 7:70–76, 1962.

71. Surgeon General. *Smoking and Health* (PHS) 79–5006. Washington, U.S. Department of Health, Education and Welfare, 1979.

72. Kafka, F. A country doctor. In: *The Basic Kafka.* New York, Pocket Books, 1979.

73. Comaroff, J. A bitter pill to swallow: placebo therapy in general practice. *Sociol Rev* 24:79–96, 1976.

74. Regier, D. A., Goldbert, I. D. and Taube, C. A. The de facto U.S. mental health services system. *Arch Gen Psychiat* 35:685–693, 1978.

75. Ebert, R. Cited in Bishop, J. M. Infuriating tensions: science and the medical student. *J Med Educ* 59:91–102, 1984.

76. Berrien, R. What future for primary care private practice? *New Eng J Med* 316:334–337, 1987.

77. Eisenberg, L. Health care: for patients or for profits? *Amer J Psychiat* 143:1015–1019, 1986.

78. Jonsen, A. R. Leadership in meeting ethical challenges. *J Med Educ* 62:95–99, 1987.

Through Clinical Method To a More Humane Medicine

by

I. R. McWhinney, M.D.

Method is central to any scholarly or professional discipline. Be it history or archaeology, physics or neurology, mastery of the discipline requires mastery of a method, techniques for gathering information and rules for classifying information and validating evidence. Implicit in the method are assumptions about the objectives of the method and the information that is relevant.

A discipline's method is not static. It evolves under the influence of changes in knowledge and, in the case of applied disciplines, changes in objectives. For over a hundred years, medicine has been served by a clinical method (I will call it the traditional method) that has proved extraordinarily effective in meeting certain objectives. However, there is now mounting evidence that this method is inadequate to meet the needs of the late twentieth century.

The Origins of the Traditional Clinical Method

The traditional method originated in France at the turn of the nineteenth century. Up to that time, medicine lacked a clinical method and a nosology that was universally accepted as useful. Sydenham, it is true, had demonstrated the predictive power of a nosology based on observations of the natural history of disease;[1] however, the nosologies of his eighteenth century successors did not have this power; they were "uncorrelated catalogues of clinical manifestations . . . lacking the prognostic or anatomic significance that would make the results practical or useful."

All this changed in early nineteenth century France, when clinicians began to turn their attention to the physical examination of the patient. New instruments such as the Laennec stethoscope revealed a new range of clinical information. At the same time, clinicians began to describe the morbid anatomy of the internal organs after death and to correlate physical signs with post-mortem appearances. These two changes went hand in hand. According to Foucault,[2] "The constitution of pathological anatomy at the period when the clinicians were defining their method is no mere coincidence: the balance of experience required that the gaze directed on the individual and the language of description should rest upon the stable, visible, legible basis of death." The result was a radically new classification of disease based on morbid anatomy, a far more powerful classification system than the nosologies of the eighteenth century.

English physicians, who had displayed little enthusiasm for the botanical classifications of the eighteenth century, become so convinced by the French clinico-pathologists that, according to Crookshank,[3] "to interpret in terms of specific diseases [became] almost the only duty of the diagnostician."

This change was not merely an advance in medical knowledge: it was a change in the way sick people were perceived. "It meant that the relation between the visible and the invisible. . . . changed its structure, revealing through gaze and language what had previously been below and beyond their domain."[2] The change involved "a reorganization of the elements that make up the pathological phenomenon [a grammar of signs has replaced a botany of symptoms], a definition of a linear series of morbid events, [as opposed to the table of nosological species], a welding of the disease onto the organism."[2]

This transformation was the beginning of the modern era in medicine. Certain social changes were necessary for the new medicine to become possible: "a reorganization of the hospital field, a new definition of the status of the patient in society, and the establishment of a certain relationship between public assistance and medical experience, between help and knowledge."[2] The reorganization of the hospitals and medical schools in the wake of the French Revolution prepared the ground for "a mutation in medical knowledge".[2]

The emergence of the method has been described by Tait,[4] who studied the archives of the clinical records of St. Bartholomew's Hospital in London, England. In the early nineteenth century, case notes were an unstructured account of the patient's complaints and the physician's superficial observations. By the 1820s, the stethoscope was being used, and notes on physical signs in the chest began to appear. The first part of the record to gain a regular structure, around 1850, was the post mortem report. By 1880 there had emerged a more structured method for recording the history and physical examination that resembled the modern form. Thus, the process that had begun in late eighteenth century France culminated a century later in a fully defined clinical method.

Advances in investigative technology have greatly increased the precision of the method, and advances in microbiology, physiology, and biochemistry have increased its power to make causal inferences. The method's aim, however, is still to interpret symptoms and signs in terms of physical pathologic findings. This is both its greatest strength and severest limitation.

The strength of the method lies in two of its features. First, it tells the clinicians precisely what they have to do to get the required results: "Take the patient's history and conduct the examination and investigation in the prescribed way, and you will either arrive at the pathological diagnosis or be able to exclude organic disease." No clinical method had done this before. Second, it provides precise criteria for validation. The pathologist tells the clinician whether he is right or wrong. The great powers of inference and prediction conferred by the method not only led to its dominance in medical thought but also paved the way for the great advances of technological medicine in this century.

LIMITATIONS OF THE TRADITIONAL METHOD

The traditional method is strictly objective. Its aim is to diagnose a disease rather than to understand a patient. It does not aim, in any systematic way, to understand the meaning of the illness for the patient or to place it in the context of the patient's biography or culture. It is not designed to deal with the moral and spiritual problems experienced by patients. Subjective matters, such as feelings and relationships, are excluded from consideration; the physician is encouraged to be objective and detached. The objectivity of the traditional method fits well with its nineteenth cen-

tury origins; it is, indeed, a product of the European Enlighten-
ment.

Paradoxically, it is the successes of medical technology that
have exposed so vividly the limitations of the traditional
method. Concentration on the technical aspects of care has di-
verted us from the patient's inner world, an aspect of illness the
method does not routinely force on our attention. The complexities and discomforts of modern therapeutics have made it even
more important for us to understand the patient's experience.
Our neglect of this may explain the remarkable increase in the
number of books and articles written by patients about their illnesses. Many of these articles have been critical of the care the
patients received.[5] Articles written by physicians or their rela-
tives are of special interest, for they often identify very vividly
the defects of the method. A recent example is Sacks' description
of his experience following a mountaineering accident.[6] Sacks, a
neurologist, concludes that the classic neurologic method is not
adequate for understanding the experiences of patients.

One poignant example of the genre is the account by a physician of his own experience with slowly progressive macular
degeneration.[7] "Through all of these years," he writes, "and despite many encounters with skilled and experienced professionals, no ophthalmologist has at any time suggested any devices
that might be of assistance to me. No ophthalmologist has mentioned any of the many ways in which I could stem the deterio-
ration in the quality of my life. Fortunately, I have discovered a
number of means whereby I have helped myself, and the purpose of this essay is to call the attention of the ophthalmological
world to some of these devices and courteously but firmly, to
complain of what appears to be the ophthalmologists' attitude:
We are interested in vision but have little interest in blindness."
This example should not be taken as a criticism of ophthalmol-
ogy. The ophthalmologists were only applying the traditional
method, according to which macular degeneration is relevant
and the experience of blindness is not.

Criticism of our clinical method is also to be found in the literature on doctor-patient communication.[8] All too frequently
we do not listen to our patients, perceive their needs, or under-

archy: the milieu interieur, the person and the interpersonal level. Systems theory has its roots in engineering, cybernetics, Gestalt psychology, and operations research. The method of nineteenth century science was to deal with problems by "cutting them down to size," separating them from their surroundings and reducing them as far as possible to linear causal chains. Systems theory seeks to do the opposite: enlarge the problems until all their significant relationships are included.

Although the biopsychosocial model has been widely accepted conceptually, there are still influential physicians who oppose any departure from the biomedical model.[14] I think, however, that these often miss the point. Those who accept the biopsychosocial model do not do so because it pushes back the boundaries of medicine to include personal maladjustments and social conflicts. They accept it because people with diseases like cancer, heart disease, multiple sclerosis and macular degeneration have a deep yearning to be understood.

FROM MODEL TO METHOD

The biopsychosocial model provides us with a powerful theory of illness. It is one thing, however, to have a theory of illness and another to express it in the form of a clinical method. In order to have a practical outcome, a new theory of illness must result in a new clinical method. It is, I believe, our inattention to this fact that has stultified efforts to reform medical practice and the medical school curriculum. Our attempts at curriculum reform often starts from the wrong end. We ask ourselves, "What courses should we add to the curriculum? Psychology? Sociology? Anthropology?" We add courses on interviewing to the teaching of clinical methods without changing the method itself. These efforts are doomed to failure unless they are accompanied by a clinical method that demands the use of these skills and this knowledge. We need to start at the other end, by developing first a transformed clinical method. Once this is achieved, the rest will follow. It will soon become clear what courses, if any, must be added to the curriculum, and what additional skills must be learned.

If I understand Foucault rightly, the modern method did not begin with pathological anatomy. It began with a clinical method. It was from the vantage point of a new clinical method that Bichat looked with a new vision on a field of knowledge that already existed. The new clinical data gave new meaning to the already existing practice of necropsy. Similarly with Flexner. By the time of the Flexner report, the modern clinical method was fully defined. The means already existed for applying the new physical sciences which were to be incorporated into the curriculum.

A Patient-Centered Clinical Method

It is against this theoretical background that the doctor-patient communication group at Western have been developing and testing a new clinical method.[15,16] We have called it a patient-centered method (not a new name), because it aims to understand the meaning of the illness for the patient as well as to diagnose his disease. We wanted the method to have the same features as the traditional method: to give the physician a clear injunction, and to provide precise criteria for validation.

Like the traditional method, the patient-centered method reduces and simplifies. At the same time, it does not deal in abstractions. It sets out to understand the patient's concrete experiences. The physician is enjoined to discover the patient's expectations, his feelings about the illness, and his fears. He does this by trying to enter the patient's world and to see the illness through the patient's eyes. The physician using the patient-centered method invites and encourages openness and expression of feeling by the patient. Expectations, feelings and fears are often not made explicit, but expressed in the form of subtle cues, which will be picked up only if the physician is listening with great attention.

The method is validated by both process and outcome assessments. Our first step was to produce precise definitions of cues to expectations, feelings and fears. We also defined a "prompt" as a signal from the patient that his expectations, feelings or fears have not been acknowledged. This often takes the form of a restatement of the original problem cue. The next was to develop criteria for the physician's response to a cue. We defined four: facilitating behavior (any verbal comment that encourages the patient to express himself), acknowledgments (any verbal expression that indicates that the patient has been heard), cut-offs (failure to respond to a cue, e.g., by interrupting or changing the subject), and returns, in which the physician remedies a previous cut-off or lack of acknowledgment by reopening the topic. We were then able to train observers to score the cues and responses in a videotape or audiotape of a doctor-patient encounter, and to attain a high level of inter-observer reliability. Using this instrument, we have been able to demonstrate an increasing degree of "patient-centeredness" in family medicine residents at different stages of their training.[17]

In the outcome assessment, the patient is interviewed to ascertain to what extent the doctor has understood and dealt with the patient's expectations, feelings and fears. It could be objected that patients are not good judges of a physician's performance. Although this may be true of the physician's clinical competence, I would argue that patients are very good judges of whether their concerns have been acknowledged and listened to. Of course, the patient-centered method must also show clinical competence. To this end, we include in our instrument an assessment of the physician's clinical performance.

One of our graduate students studied 73 adult patients with one new symptom presenting to six family physicians.[18] He found that a high score for patient-centeredness was related to decreased patient concern about the presenting symptom, a perception by the patient that the presenting problem was fully discussed, and a perception that his reason for visiting had been fully understood by the doctor. The patient-centered consultations were related neither to high nor low scores for clinical competence.

Does Patient-Centeredness Influence Healing?

So far, we have not used our instrument to investigate recovery from illness. We have, however, some interesting data from other studies. In a study of the natural history of headache in patients presenting to family physicians,[19] we found unexpectedly that the strongest predictor of recovery from the headache a year later, was the patients' statements, shortly after their first visit, that they had had good opportunity to discuss their problem with the doctor.

In another study from our own department, Martin Bass and colleagues[20] interviewed patients one month and three months after a visit to a family doctor with a new symptom. The factor most strongly associated with recovery at one month was the patient's complete agreement with the doctor's opinion.

Approaching patient-centeredness from another angle, Greenfield and his colleagues[21] coached patients to ask questions and negotiate medical decisions with their physicians. When compared with a control group receiving a standard educational session, these patients were more involved in the interaction with the physician and were twice as effective in obtaining information from the physician. They also reported fewer limitations in physical activities due to their disease.

ART AND TECHNIQUE

Some of our critics have maintained that humanism in medicine cannot—and should not—be reduced to a technique. To this I reply that medicine is an art and that all artists make use of techniques and formulas. Even in prayer and meditation (the art of arts) techniques are described. In his book *Art and Illusion*, Ernst Gombrich[22] describes how painters use a formula for drawing the human head. Constable had a formula for painting clouds— remarkably similar to the scientist's classification of clouds. Of course, this is only a beginning. Having used a formula for sketching out the basic features of the human head, the artist then proceeds to use his creative talent to flesh out the portrait in all its individuality.

Similarly with our method. The technique is only a beginning. The attainment of a full "picture" of the patient requires of the physician all that he has, as a person and as a clinician. Once he begins to practice in this way, he soon encounters some very difficult and even disturbing questions. The traditional clinical method, with its short questions and answers, and its avoidance of feeling, tends to protect us from questions like these. Once they begin to teach the patient-centered method, teachers soon learn that they also have to deal with its personal consequences. Students are no longer sheltered from confronting their own inadequacies in meeting patients' needs. This very confrontation is itself an opportunity for the growth of self-knowledge and maturity in the physician. Thus, if properly used, the method leads to a different kind of teaching. It becomes learner-centered.

Consequences for Medical Education

In his book *Science and the Modern World*, A. N. Whitehead[23] has expressed with great clarity what is wrong with modern professional education. "Professional education," said Whitehead, "produces minds in a groove. Now to be mentally in a groove is to live in contemplating a given set of abstractions. The groove prevents straying across country, and the abstraction abstracts from something to which no further attention is paid. But there is no groove of abstraction which is adequate for the comprehension of human life. Thus, in the modern world, the celibacy of the medieval learned class has been replaced by the celibacy of the intellect which is divorced from the concrete contemplation of the complete facts." "We are left," says Whitehead, "with no expansion of wisdom and with greater need of it." I would go further and say that wisdom is declining in the modern world.

In discussing the remedy, Whitehead is critical of our preoccupation with intellectual analysis. He fears that, in our attempts to attain a balanced development, we will supplement professional training (the mastery of a set of abstractions) with a slighter study of a different set of abstractions. This could so easily happen if we add courses in behavioral science to the curriculum. Courses in behavioral science usually deal with abstractions rather than concrete human experience. It could even happen if we add courses in the humanities, for, in the modern university, the humanities have not escaped from the pressure to analyze. In Whitehead's view, "The makeweight which balances the thoroughness of the specialist intellectual training should be of a radically different kind from purely intellectual analytical knowledge." The need is for "aesthetic education."

My thesis, then, is that medicine will not necessarily be made more humane by adding courses to the curriculum. What we need is a *transformed clinical method* that will lead us naturally into the subjective aspects of medicine. At the same time we will need to teach clinical medicine in a different way—a way that will foster, rather than stifle, the moral and aesthetic development of the student.

Let me give some examples of how this might enrich medical education. We tend to forget that medicine has a very rich imaginative and descriptive literature. Writers of genius and talent have through the ages reflected on the great themes of medicine: suffering, illness, healing, dying. As I mentioned earlier, some have given us graphic personal experiences of their own illnesses. Some have written perceptively on the life and work of a physician. Even the literature of clinical description can include the subjective experience of patients. The writings of Oliver Sacks are a modern example of this genre.[6,24] Sacks' case histories are not only good clinical histories, but testaments to the human spirit in its triumph over suffering. Medicine has its own poetry—a poetry we can all experience if we learn to listen to our patients' stories.

I can visualize a course in the medical curriculum that would sensitize students to the feelings of their patients. Students could be asked to imagine the experience of losing a pregnancy, having inoperable cancer, losing one's vision, caring for a spouse with Alzheimer's disease, bereavement, being paraplegic, and so on. They could then meet in a small group with people who had gone through these experiences, and read related clinical descriptions and imaginative literature.

If I am correct, there are far-reaching implications for medical education. If physicians are to change in the way I have suggested, their education will have to encourage reflection, personal development and the growth of self-knowledge. The current environment of the medical school, with its information overload, frenzied activity and competitive ethos, in many ways discourages personal development of this kind. Medical scientists sometimes make reference to "the frontiers of knowledge." I think they have in mind a frontier that is "out there." The newest and most challenging frontier may be within us.

REFERENCES

1. Feinstein, A. R. *Clinical Judgement.* Baltimore, Williams and Wilkins, 1967.

2. Foucault, M. *The Birth of the Clinic. An Archaeology of Medical Perception.* Translated from the French by A. M. Sheridan Smith. New York, Vintage Books, 1975.

3. Crookshank, F. G. The theory of diagnosis. *Lancet* 2:939–942, 995–999, 1926.

4. Tait, I. The History and Function of Clinical Records. Unpublished thesis for the degree of Doctor of Medicine, University of Cambridge, 1979.

5. Baker, S. S. Information Decisionmaking and the Relationship Between Client and Health Care Professional in Published Personal Narratives, D Phil dissertation, University of Texas, Dallas, 1984.

6. Sacks, O. *A Leg to Stand On.* London, Duckworth, 1984.

7. Stetten, D., Jr. Coping with blindness. *New Engl J Med* 305:458–460, 1981.

8. Ley, L. Patients' understanding and recall in clinical communication failure. In Pendleton, D., Hasler, J. (eds): *Doctor-Patient Communication.* London, *Acad Pr*, 89–107, 1983.

9. James, W. *The Varieties of Religious Experience.* New York, New American Library of World Literature, 29, 1958.

10. Wilbush, J. Climacteric symptom formation: Donovan's contribution. *Maturitas* 3:99–105, 1981.

11. Balint, M. The other part of medicine. *Lancet* 1:40–42, 1961.

12. Balint, M. *The Doctor, His Patient and the Illness*. London, Pitman Med Pub, 1964.

13. Engel, G. L. The clinical application of the biopsychosocial model. *Am J Psychiatry* 137:535–544, 1980.

14. Seldin, D. W. Presidential Address. The Boundaries of Medicine. *Trans Assoc Am Phys* 94:74–84, 1981.

15. Levenstein, J. H., McCracken, E. C., McWhinney, I. R. et al. The patient-centred clinical method. I. A model for the doctor-patient interaction in family practice. *Fam Pract* 3,1:24–30, 1986.

16. Brown, J., Stewart, M., McCracken, E. et al. The patient-centered clinical method. II. Definition and application. *Fam Pract* 3,1:75–79, 1986.

17. Stewart, M., Brown, J., Levenstein, J. et al. The patient-centered clinical method. III. Changes in residents' performance in the patient-centered clinical method over two months of training. *Fam Pract* 3,3:164–167, 1986.

18. Henbest, R. J. A study of the patient-centered approach in family practice. M. Cl. Sc. thesis, University of Western Ontario, London, 1985.

19. Bass, M. J., McWhinney, I. R., Dempsey, J. B. et al. Predictors of outcome in headache patients presenting to family physicians—a one year prospective study. *Headache J* 26,6:285–294, 1986.

20. Bass, M. J., Buck, C., Turner, L. et al. The physician's actions and the outcome of illness. *J Fam Pract* 23:43–47, 1986.

21. Greenfield, S., Kaplan, S., Ware, J. E., Jr. Expanding patient involvement in care. *Annals of Int Med* 102:520–528, 1985.

22. Gombrich, E. H. *Art and Illusion*. London, Phaidon Press, 1962.

23. Whitehead, A. N. *Science and the Modern World*. Cambridge, Cambridge University Press, 1926.

24. Sacks, O. *Awakenings*. London, Duckworth and Co., 1973.

PARTICIPANTS
CONFERENCE ON THE BIOPSYCHOSOCIAL CONCEPT
OF ILLNESS AND DISEASE

May 12–15, 1987
Wickenburg, Arizona

HARRISON ALTER, *Medical Education Consultant, Henry J. Kaiser Family Foundation, 2400 Sand Hill Road, Menlo Park, CA 94025*

CAROL A. ASCHENBRENER, M.D., *Associate Dean, Medical Student Affairs, University of Iowa College of Medicine, 100 College of Medicine, Administration Building, Iowa City, IA 52242*

HARRY N. BEATY, M.D., *Dean, Medical School, Northwestern University, 303 East Chicago Avenue, Chicago, IL 60611*

JOHN A. BENSON, JR., M.D., *President, American Board of Internal Medicine, 200 S. W. Market Street, Portland, OR 97201*

JANET BICKEL, *Staff Associate, Association of American Medical Colleges, One Dupont Circle, NW, Ste. 200, Washington, DC 20036*

DODY BIENENSTOCK, M.D., *Assistant Professor, Department of Psychiatry, Room 3G12, McMaster University School of Medicine, 1200 Main Street West, Hamilton, Ontario L8N 3Z5, Canada*

DANIEL S. BLUMENTHAL, M.D., *Chairman, Department of Community Medicine and Family Practice, Morehouse School of Medicine, 720 Westview Drive, SW, Atlanta, GA 30310–1495*

STEVEN A. COHEN-COLE, M.D., *Associate Professor of Psychiatry, Emory University School of Medicine, 1365 Clifton Road, Atlanta, GA 30322*

JACK M. COLWILL, M.D., *Chairman, Family and Community Medicine, University of Missouri, Columbia School of Medicine, One Hospital Drive, Columbia, MO 65212*

ROBERT W. P. CUTLER, M.D., *Associate Dean, Faculty Affairs and Medical Education, Stanford University School of Medicine, 300 Pasteur Drive, Stanford, CA 94305*

DOUGLAS A. DROSSMAN, M.D., *Associate Professor of Medicine/Psychiatry, Department of Medicine-Gastroenterology, University of North Carolina, Room 324, Clinical Sciences Building 229H, 901 Kings Mill Road, Chapel Hill, NC 27514*

LEON EISENBERG, M.D., *Professor and Chairman, Department of Social Medicine and Health Policy, Harvard Medical School, 25 Shattuck Street, Boston, MA 02115*

GEORGE L. ENGEL, M.D., *Professor Emeritus of Psychiatry, Professor Emeritus of Medicine, University of Rochester, Medical Center, 300 Crittenden Boulevard, Rochester, NY 14842*

ALBERTO GALOFRE, M.D., *Associate Dean for Curriculum, School of Medicine, St. Louis University, 1402 South Grand Boulevard, St. Louis, MO 63104*

DAVID S. GREER, M.D., *Dean, Medical School, Brown University, 97 Waterman Street, Providence, RI 02912*

ROBERT J. HAGGERTY, M.D., *President, W.T. Grant Foundation, 919 Third Avenue, New York, NY 10022*

CARL F. HINZ, JR., M.D., *Professor of Medicine and Associate Dean, Academic Affairs and Clinical Education, University of Connecticut, School of Medicine, Farmington, CT 06032*

THOMAS S. INUI, M.D., *Head, General Internal Medicine, University of Washington, Harborview Medical Center ZA-60, 325 Ninth Avenue, Seattle, WA 98104*

JOSEPH E. JOHNSON, III, M.D., *Dean, Medical School, University of Michigan, M7300 Medical Science Building 1, 1301 Catherine Road, Ann Arbor, MI 48109-0010*

STANLEY G. KORENMAN, M.D., *Associate Dean, Education in Medical Science, University of California at Los Angeles, School of Medicine, Los Angeles, CA 90024*

MACK LIPKIN, JR., M.D., *Director, Primary Care, Associate Professor of Medicine, New York University Medical Center Department of Medicine, 16S-New Bellevue, 550 First Ave., New York, NY 10016*

IAN R. MCWHINNEY, M.D., *Professor and Chairman, Department of Family Medicine, Kresge Building, Room K101, University of Western Ontario, London, Ontario N6A 5C1, Canada*

JACK H. MEDALIE, M.D., *Chairman, Department of Family Medicine, Case Western Reserve School of Medicine, First Floor, West Wing #165, 2119 Abington Road, Cleveland, OH 44106*

JOAN E. MORGENTHAU, M.D., *Director, Health Services, Smith College, 69 Paradise Road, Northampton, MA 01063*

DENNIS H. NOVACK, M.D., *Associate Physician, Division of General Internal Medicine, Rhode Island Hospital, 593 Eddy Street, Providence, RI 02902*

S. SCOTT OBENSHAIN, M.D., *Assistant Dean, Undergraduate Medical Education, School of Medicine, University of New Mexico, Albuquerque, NM 87131*

CHARLES E. ODEGAARD, PH.D., *President Emeritus, University of Washington, 222 Miller Hall (DQ-12), Seattle, WA 98195*

THEODORE J. PHILLIPS, M.D., *Professor, Family Medicine, Acting Dean, School of Medicine (SC-64), University of Washington, Seattle, WA 98195*

TIMOTHY E. QUILL, M.D., *Clinical Assistant Professor of Medicine, Internal Medicine Department, Genesee Hospital, 224 Alexander Street, Rochester, NY 14607*

CHRISTIAN N. RAMSEY, JR., M.D., *Professor and Chairman, Department of Family Medicine, The University of Oklahoma, Health Sciences Center, P.O. Box 26901, 800 Northeast 15th Street, Room 501, Oklahoma City, OK 73190*

PAUL G. RAMSEY, M.D., *Associate Professor, Department of Medicine (RG-20), University of Washington, Seattle, WA 98195*

REBECCA W. RIMEL, *Vice President, Pew Charitable Trusts, 3 Parkway, Ste. 501, Philadelphia, PA 19102-1305*

DAVID SATCHER, M.D., PH.D., *President, Meharry Medical College, School of Medicine, 1005 D. B. Todd, Jr. Boulevard, Nashville, TN 37208*

JUDY SCHMICKLEY, *Meeting Coordinator, Henry J. Kaiser Family Foundation, 2400 Sand Hill Road, Menlo Park, CA 94025*

EDWARD L. SCHOR, M.D., *Program Officer, Henry J. Kaiser Family Foundation, 2400 Sand Hill Road, Menlo Park, CA 94025*

MICHAEL A. SCHWARTZ, M.D., *Associate Professor of Clinical Psychiatry, New York Medical College, St. Vincent's Hospital and Medical Center of New York, 203 W. 12th Street, Room 606, New York, NY 10011*

HENRY M. SEIDEL, M.D., *Associate Dean for Student Affairs, Johns Hopkins School of Medicine, 720 Rutland Avenue, Baltimore, MD 21205*

ROBERT C. SMITH, M.D., *Associate Professor of Medicine and Psychiatry, Michigan State University, B220 Life Sciences Building, East Lansing, MI 48824*

G. GAYLE STEPHENS, M.D., *Professor of Family Practice, University of Alabama, University Station, Birmingham, AL 35294*

PAULA L. STILLMAN, M.D., *Associate Dean for Curriculum, University of Massachusetts Medical School, 55 Lake Avenue North, Worcester, MA 01605*

ALVIN R. TARLOV, M.D. *President, Henry J. Kaiser Family Foundation, 2400 Sand Hill Road, Menlo Park, CA 94025*

ROBERT H. WALDMAN, M.D., *Dean, College of Medicine, University of Nebraska, 42nd Street and Dewey Avenue, Omaha, NE 68105*

RALPH O. WALLERSTEIN, M.D., *Clinical Professor of Medicine, School of Medicine, University of California, San Francisco, 3838 California Street, San Francisco, CA 94118*

KERR L. WHITE, M.D., *Retired Deputy Director Health Sciences, Rockefeller Foundation, Rte. 1, Box 285, State Road 674, Stanardsville, VA 22973*

OSBORNE P. WIGGINS, PH.D., *Assistant Professor, Department of Philosophy, Graduate Faculty of Political and Social Science, New School for Social Research, 65 Fifth Avenue, New York, NY 10003*